PRACTICAL GUIDE TO

OCCUPATIONAL
HEALTH AND SAFETY

PRACTICAL GUIDE TO

OCCUPATIONAL

HEALTH AND SAFETY

PAUL A. ERICKSON

Occupational and Environmental
Health and Safety Program
Anna Maria College
Paxton, Massachusetts

ACADEMIC PRESS

San Diego   New York   Boston   London   Sydney   Tokyo   Toronto

Find Us on the Web! http://www.apnet.com

This book is printed on acid-free paper. ∞

Copyright © 1996 by ACADEMIC PRESS, INC.

Academic Press, Inc.
A Division of Harcourt Brace & Company
525 B Street, Suite 1900, San Diego, California 92101-4495

United Kingdom Edition published by
Academic Press Limited
24-28 Oval Road, London NW1 7DX

Library of Congress Cataloging-in-Publication Data

Erickson, Paul A.
    Practical guide to occupational health and safety / by Paul A.
    Erickson.
            p.   cm.
    Includes index.
    ISBN 0-12-240570-6 (alk. paper)
    1. Industrial hygiene--Handbooks, manuals, etc. 2. Industrial
safety--Handbooks, manuals, etc.   I. Title.
RC967.E685   1996
658.3'82--dc20   96-7675
                                                  CIP

PRINTED IN THE UNITED STATES OF AMERICA
96 97 98 99 00 01 EB 9 8 7 6 5 4 3 2 1

For
Dr. Donald G. Erickson
with admiration and love

CONTENTS

HEALTH AND SAFETY PROGRAMS

PART III

SPECIAL ISSUES

PREFACE

The professional literature on occupational health and safety encompasses a wide range of specialties of interest to diverse audiences, including laboratory managers, loss control managers, industrial hygienists, corporate insurance underwriters, medical services personnel, and human resource managers. However, there is a clear need for a highly integrative book that focuses on both the conceptual and the practical informational needs of the industrial compliance officer and other workplace practitioners who, while having daily responsibility for the health and safety of employees, have little formal training in the relevant specialties. This book is intended to meet that need. It is also intended for use as an introductory text for graduate students enrolled in occupational or environmental health and safety programs or in specialized business management programs that increasingly give emphasis to the role of health and safety in corporate decision-making.

Today, any book that would purport to provide both a conceptual and a practical overview of the field of occupational health and safety must include consideration of not only the scientific and technical aspects of health and safety risks, but also the legal, economic, ethical, and business ramifications of the management of those risks. Moreover, all of these considerations must be addressed in light of the realities of the modern workplace in terms of the yet developing global economy and highly sophisticated information technology.

In order to achieve an appropriately balanced conceptual and practical treatment of the many aspects of contemporary occupational health and safety, I have divided this book into three parts.

Part 1 presents a broad overview of the field, with particular emphasis on national and international factors that influence the practical application of health and safety principles in an industrial setting. In this section, the scientific, technical, and managerial aspects of hazard and risk assessment, the use of occupational health and safety standards, and in-plant audits are given particular emphasis.

Part 2 focuses on the design and implementation of various types of in-plant programs that are the basic means for ensuring corporate compliance with selected health and safety regulations. The selection of specific regulations for inclusion in this section primarily reflects their relevance to a broad diversity of industries and, in some instances, to particular issues that are likely to influence the practice of industrial hygiene in industry at large for many years to come.

Part 3 deals with special issues that extend well beyond the jurisdictional interests of any individual regulation and typically require a comprehensive appreciation of the need for a holistic integration of workplace health and safety with developing issues in science, technology, and business management.

For both the design and the preparation of this book I am indebted to many persons, in particular to the J. William Fulbright Foreign Scholarship Board and the U.S. Information Agency for a Fulbright award that allowed me to spend several months in Malaysia and thereby further develop the international context of this book; Dr. Halim Shafie and Dr. Hashim Hassan, Director and Deputy Director of the Malaysian National Institute of Public Administration (INTAN), who graciously provided me with a thoroughly professional setting for exploring occupational health and safety programs throughout Southeast Asia; Augustine Koh Oon Shing of INTAN, for his masterful guidance in the intricacies of integrated environmental planning and management and their relevance to occupational health and safety; Dr. Lee Chee San for his thoughtful critique of my original outline of this book; Jean Letendre, Bonnie Thornton, Dr. David Barnes, and Dr. R. Burt Prater, Jr., who provided me with key technical information; Hans Ahlgren, Richard Johnson, and Brant Sayre, for the privilege of working with them to implement comprehensive health and safety programs; and Claire (Myers) Erickson, for those technical, scientific, and editorial skills that she has made available to me throughout the development of this book.

PART I

OVERVIEW OF OCCUPATIONAL HEALTH AND SAFETY

CHAPTER I

SCOPE OF OCCUPATIONAL HEALTH AND SAFETY

HOLISTIC APPROACH

In the continually expanding context of occupational health and safety, the word *safety* denotes concern for *physical injuries* that might be experienced by the worker, such as cuts, abrasions, punctures, burns, and the crushing of feet or arms; *health*, for those *physiological injuries* that are typically associated with illness and debilitation caused by exposure to chemical toxins or infectious biological agents; *welfare*, for a range of *psychological conditions*, including stress and "burn out," which may derive from or be exacerbated by workplace conditions. In contemporary industry, the word safety (especially as it might be used in a job title, such as "safety officer," or as an objective, as in "safety is everyone's responsibility") is generally understood to denote worker health and welfare as well as safety—a meaning that will be used throughout this text.

While the terms safety, health, and welfare are useful for differentiating among broad categories of work-related injuries as well as different regulatory requirements that may pertain to those injuries, they are perhaps most useful for defining the dimensions of the contemporary approach to risk management in the workplace—an approach that, by recognizing the interconnected physical, physiological, and psychological dimensions of human well-being, promotes a holistic appreciation of the worker's well-being and a comprehensive understanding of just how workplace conditions contribute to or detract from it.

As shown in Figure 1.1, the contemporary holistic appreciation of worker safety is inclusive not only of the physical, physiological, and psychological dimensions of the human being, and not only of direct workplace exposure to hazards, but also of environmental exposures that occur outside

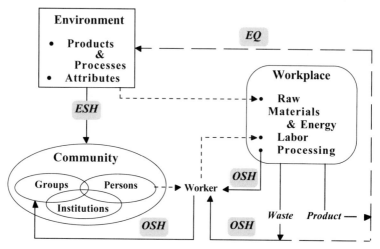

FIGURE I.I   A holistic overview of the workplace, environmental quality, and the human community. Shaded acronyms include historically distinct areas of study; EQ, environmental quality; OSH, occupational safety and health; and ESH, environmental safety and health. Sometimes referred to as the "product cycle," such a diagram emphasizes the arbitrariness of historical distinctions among the various mechanisms that influence human health and safety.

of the workplace. Thus the worker cannot be defined solely by workplace experience, but is defined by the worker's experience in the broader social community and the environment that envelops that community. In this sense, it is increasingly difficult (if not irrelevant) to differentiate between *occupational health* and *environmental health*, or even *human health* from *environmental quality*. Today, the worker's well-being as a real-world integration of a person's total life experience must be the focus.

This perspective of worker health and safety is central to a paradigm that was essentially formulated by the United Nations Conference on Environment and Development (UNCED), commonly known as the Earth Summit (Rio, 1992). This paradigm, often referred to as the "Integrated Environmental Planning and Management" paradigm, is based on a broad consensus that the management of human health and safety and the management of environmental quality can be carried out more efficiently when both efforts are integrated. This consensus is expressed in the 1992 U.N. Earth Summit Agenda and has broad social ramifications for both public and private decision making:

> The primary need is to integrate environmental and developmental decision-making processes. To do this, governments should conduct a national review and, where appropriate, improve the processes of decision-making so

as to achieve the progressive integration of economic, social, and environmental issues in the pursuit of development that is economically efficient, socially equitable and responsible, and environmentally sound. (1992 Earth Summit Agenda 21, p. 66).

The acronym HSE (i.e., health, safety, environment) is frequently used in the international literature to denote the paradigm of Integrated Environmental Planning and Management. While the terms *occupational health and safety* and *environmental health and safety* are still commonly used to focus, respectively, on workplace and nonworkplace contributions to human health and safety, it is widely understood that such a distinction may often obscure rather than clarify the dynamic linkage between environmental processes and attributes, human activities (e.g., work), and human health and safety.

CORPORATE RESPONSIBILITY

At both national and international levels, the modern corporation is perceived as having both a moral and a legal responsibility to protect its employees from (a) workplace sources of injury and (b) workplace insults to a worker's preexisting debilitation. While the degree of responsibility and the extent of afforded protection is certainly subject to ongoing social and legal debate, no modern corporation can reasonably expect to prosper without elevating its concern for worker health and safety to a level commensurate with such historic corporate concerns as the availability of raw materials, production costs, marketing, and loss control. In relatively large companies (e.g., more than several hundred employees), worker health and safety often becomes the assigned responsibility of a full-time safety officer; in smaller companies, the various duties associated with a safety officer are most often performed by a number of employees who, nonetheless, have other responsibilities in production or administration.

There are many variants among organizational structures that companies use to manage workplace health and safety risks. For example, functions that pertain to worker safety and which are also identified in specific regulations, such as those associated with a "hazardous waste coordinator" or "laboratory hygiene officer," may be assigned to supervisors of those departments having primary operational responsibility for complying with a particular regulation. The maintenance supervisor is, therefore, often designated as the hazardous waste coordinator; the laboratory supervisor as the laboratory hygiene officer. However, some companies may find it preferable to assign these same functions to a human resources officer.

Because of the increasing number of regulations that directly or indirectly pertain to occupational health and safety, and because of the increasing interconnectedness of these regulations, it is important that corporate responsibility and authority regarding the management of workplace risks are most usefully consolidated in a committee that reflects all dimensions of both worker health and corporate responsibility.

Ideally, a corporate risk management committee would consist of at least (a) corporate executive(s), (b) safety officer, (c) key supervisors/managers, (d) corporate legal counsel, (e) human resources officer, and (f) workforce representatives.

It is through such a committee that the safety officer (or, in the absence of a safety officer, other key supervisors/managers having responsibility for workplace safety) is able to avoid all too common problems, including:

- Lack of sufficient authority to implement safety-related changes at the department level,
- Isolation from higher level decision makers who, knowingly or unknowingly, must bear the potential legal liability associated with workplace injury, and
- Isolation from production-level personnel who, despite their primary responsibility for production, also play a crucial role in the implementation of an effective safety program.

COMMENSURATE RESPONSIBILITY AND AUTHORITY

The modern management of workplace health and safety is essentially proactive. It requires that priority be given to the recognition of potential hazards and risks and, therefore, to alternative means for minimizing those potentials. All too often, however, there is little correlation between corporate responsibility and corporate authority—a situation that results in potential hazards and risks becoming actual emergencies.

For example, a safety officer may determine that the on-site inventory of a particularly hazardous chemical is several times larger than is needed for quarterly production purposes. The storage of the excess inventory presents a demonstrable risk not only to employees but also to the surrounding community. It may well be that the primary reason for the excess inventory is that the company's purchasing agents are ever alert to the economic advantage to buying in bulk . . . regardless of production needs. While the safety officer has responsibility for minimizing chemical hazards and risks, the safety officer typically has no authority regarding the policies of the purchasing department that create the hazard and risk.

Historically derived "chains-of-command," "areas" of responsibility, and "job descriptions" typically militate against a modern holistic approach to workplace health and safety and must be reassessed to ensure that those who have the responsibility for workplace health and safety also have an authority that is commensurate with that responsibility. This does not mean that the safety officer must be granted the powers of a chief executive, but it does mean that the safety officer must have direct access to those powers.

CORPORATE AND PERSONAL LIABILITY

The concern for worker health and safety is no longer simply a national issue; it is a concern that is central to the developing global economy—a concern that, fostered by two decades of regulatory emphasis in developed nations, is of at least equal import in developing nations. Certainly the question of the precise limits of corporate and personal liability with regard to workplace health and safety is to be answered in terms of the legal precepts and institutions of individual nations. However, there can be no question that, worldwide, governments are increasingly imposing civil and even criminal liabilities on corporations and on individual corporate executives and other key employees for failures to ensure the health and safety of employees.

Whether under the aegis of the International Standards Organization (ISO), the European Community Eco-Audit Regulation, the Canadian Standards Association, the American Society for Quality Control, the International Chamber of Commerce, the Malaysian Integrated Environmental Planning and Management Program, or any number of other international, regional, and national programs, standards and policies, the management of workplace health and safety today implies *accountability of both the corporation and the person*—moral accountability, economic accountability, and legal accountability.

The international insistence on legal accountability regarding HSE is clearly expressed in the 1992 U.N. Earth Summit Agenda:

> States shall develop national law regarding liability and compensation for the victims of pollution and other environmental damage. States shall also cooperate in an expeditious and more determined manner to develop further international law regarding liability and compensation for adverse effects of environmental damage caused by activities within their jurisdiction or control to areas beyond their jurisdiction. (1992 Earth Summit Agenda 21, Principle 13).

In the United States, legal accountability for worker health and safety has long been manifest in regulatory liabilities that result in fines levied against a corporation. In the past decade, federal and state regulations regarding worker health and safety have become more numerous and complex, and corresponding fines for noncompliance have become steadily more severe. At the same time, criminal law has increasingly been used to hold corporate owners, executives, and even floor supervisors accountable for worker health and safety. Finally, tort law has been greatly expanded, with the result that American workers have relatively easy access to the courts regarding work-related injury and illness.

The American experience regarding legal accountability for worker health and safety is paralleled by the experience of many other nations, the primary differences being those related to differences in legal systems, including differences in procedures in administrative law, differences regarding common law and civil law traditions, and differences regarding the jurisdiction of cultural and religious traditions, as in the Law of Islam.

THE WORKPLACE: NEW IMAGE FOR A NEW CENTURY

The hallmark of the industrial revolution in England is dated 1769, the year that James Watt invented the steam engine. This is not to say, of course, that the industrial revolution, which was essentially the substitution of an urban, factory-based economy for an agriculture-based economy, was established everywhere at that particular time. It took from the mid-18th century to the mid-19th century for industrialization to spread from England to Europe and the United States and to the beginning of the 20th century to extend to Asia. Industrialization is yet a new development in many parts of the world.

The hallmark of governmental regulation of the industrial workplace in the United States is dated 1970, the year that Congress created the Occupational Safety and Health Administration (OSHA), which establishes and enforces workplace health and safety standards, and the National Institute for Occupational Safety and Health (NIOSH), which conducts research on workplace health and safety standards.

Certainly there were organized attempts to prevent industrial accidents prior to 1970 in the United States and in other nations. For example, by the latter part of the 19th century and into the early 20th century, insurance companies enforced fire and safety standards, and legislatures in Germany, Great Britain, and the United States enacted specific legislation that defined the financial responsibility of corporations for injured factory workers. In addition to physical injuries, workplace-related illnesses were also recognized early in the industrial revolution, including such diseases as lung disease among miners and potters (exposed to silica dust), scrotal skin cancer among chimney sweeps (exposed to soot), neurological diseases among potters (exposed to lead glazes) and hatters (exposed to mercury), and bone disease among matchmakers (exposed to phosphorus).

While there are numerous examples of both early recognition of safety and health hazards attendant to industrialization and early attempts to regulate those hazards (e.g., Workmen's Compensation Laws, Metal and Nonmetallic Mine Safety Act, Coal Mine Health and Safety Act, Construction Safety Act), the fact remains that the vast majority of laws in the United States related to workplace health and safety have been enacted since 1960.

In short, a comprehensive and coordinated national legislative effort on behalf of worker health and safety has existed in the United States for about the last 25 years of roughly a 130-year period of national industrial development, which is approximately only the latter 19% of the duration of the American industrial revolution.

Historians and political scientists may well argue as to the relative influence of a wide range of factors that played a role in the achievement of a national commitment to worker health and safety, including the influence of the relative costs of worker compensation and workplace improvement, labor shortages during worldwide and regional wars, and the various successes and failures of the American labor movement. However, it is of particular interest to note that the major legislative efforts regarding worker health and safety essentially began with the advent of the *global village* and have continued in pace with an increasingly pervasive communications technology into the present era of a nascent *global economy*.

Throughout the past 30 years, miners in a distant state killed by a cave-in have not been simply a statistic printed in our local newspaper; through television, we have seen and heard the grief of their families and friends; and in seeing and thereby sharing their grief, we have also seen and shared their anger that the accident might, after all, have been prevented. So it is, with each accident, injury, or illness that television daily depicts and explores, that we learn what every member of any village must always learn: what happens to one can happen to another; what happens to *you* can happen to *me*.

Whether it is an industrial poisoning of an entire population, the progressive disease of a former President, the fatal addiction of a famous entertainer, the botched medical treatment of a well known newspaper reporter, or any other most recent example of human vulnerability to both natural and human-caused hazard, the instantaneous communication of that vulnerability transforms personal tragedy into communal anxiety if not outright fear. It makes no difference if a particular personal tragedy is experienced by somebody in our own city or state or even country. Should a condominium collapse in Kuala Lumpur, Malaysia, it is eminently reasonable for a condominium dweller in Boston, Massachusetts, to wonder if it can also happen there—and, if so, what can be done about it. Should an agricultural worker in California develop skin cancer as a result of exposure to a particular pesticide, it is eminently reasonable for a mother in India to wonder if her children are similarly vulnerable to a certain household pesticide—and, if so, what can be done about it.

The advent of the global village enhanced our ability to identify the types of risks and hazards we might encounter if only because others in our own village (be it town, state, or country) had already encountered them. As that global village has electronically expanded to encompass a global economy, all human experience of risks and hazards is available for what it can tell us about our own personal health and safety.

While it is premature to define all the lessons to be gleaned through a global perspective of human health and safety, it is clearly appropriate to identify relatively simple lessons learned to date that may well be considered as basic principles of a holistic approach to workplace health and safety:

1. The health and safety of a worker is influenced not only by conditions of the workplace, but also by non-work-related factors that can nonetheless be exacerbated or potentiated by the workplace.

The same workplace may present different health and safety risks to workers performing similar tasks, depending upon a wide range of personal factors, including gender, age, preexisting medical condition, genetic predisposition, physiological condition, pregnancy and reproductive potential, and substance dependence. The unequal distribution of risks within a population performing the same tasks necessarily elevates *social* (or *environmental*) *equity* to a fundamental ethical (and often legal) consideration in any modern program for managing workplace risks. It should also be noted that the question of equity is not only of ethical or legal import. For example, it is increasingly recognized that social inequities regarding nutrition and general health also have direct relevance to both the genesis and the distribution of various types of infectious diseases.

A second issue encompassed by this principle is that of *synergy*—the interaction of two or more agents so that their combined effect is greater than the sum of their individual effects. This is a particularly difficult phenomenon to manage because of our basic lack of scientific data. For example, approximately 60,000 different chemicals are in daily use in any developed society. We simply do not have data on the possible synergistic interactions among all the possible combinations of these chemicals.

2. Workplace effects on human health and safety are not restricted to either the on-site workplace or the worker.

There are basically two aspects to this principle: (a) the impacts of workplace wastes (including both the material and energetic wastes of production [i.e., direct wastes] and the wastes generated by the use and disposal of products [i.e., indirect wastes]) on environmental quality, with consequent impact on community (and therefore worker) health and safety, and (b) so-called "carry home contamination," which includes a diverse assemblage of mechanisms whereby a worker "carries" workplace-derived contaminants (e.g., asbestos dust) out of the workplace and into the home or other surroundings.

More recently, this principle gives emphasis to concerns regarding the relationship between clear-cutting virgin forests (e.g., primary growth rainforest) and the subsequent release of potential disease vectors (e.g., the carrier of Ebola virus) into a broader environment. In this sense, the workplace is defined as the logging camp or whatever facility or project results in the release of the disease vector.

THE WORKER: FIRST, A PERSON

The holistic approach to occupational health and safety is based on the understanding that any person's health and safety is a real-world integration of that person's total life experience, beginning with a specific genetic endowment and progressing along a unique continuum of events, conditions, and circumstances. The workplace is only one aspect of that continuum, just as a home is only one aspect, as is a place of recreation, a place of study, and a place of worship. We are assigned (or assign ourselves) a variety of names, such as worshiper, student, race car driver, current resident, and worker for being in such places and for doing whatever is to be done in each. However, none of these names define us utterly. We are, first and foremost, persons.

The modern discipline of occupational health and safety deals, first, with persons. It attempts to discover how the workplace can put the health and safety of persons at risk and to devise means for minimizing that risk.

Some of the persons that a workplace may put at risk are the workers in that workplace. Of these, some are at greater or lesser risk, depending upon personal factors and their specific jobs. However, regardless of the specific job or personal susceptibilities or propensities, direct workplace impacts on a worker's health or safety may result in impacts on the health and safety of other persons, including co-workers (e.g., as when chemical fumes depress the central nervous system of one worker whose subsequent physical discoordination results in a co-worker's injury), their unborn children (e.g., fetal damage, developmental injury, mutation), and other members of the broader community (e.g., workplace disease or contamination "carried" home by the worker).

Of course, the workplace can affect the health and safety of the broader community without the personal mediation of workers, as through the contamination of soil, air, and water with chemical wastes, the risk of explosion, and the generation of toxic gases.

For the larger part of the industrial revolution, the health and safety of the worker was essentially ignored; the worker was considered little more than an organic tool used for production and as easily replaced as any inanimate tool. Even with the extensive development of occupational health and safety laws and standards over the past several decades, the approach has been to deal with the worker as (in effect) a class or category, as in "blue collar laborer," "secretary," or "laboratory technician." This categorical perspective of the worker as someone defined by a specific task, a specific schedule, and a specific workplace is not sufficiently comprehensive for the rapidly developing, holistic, approach to environmental and human health management.

While there is international consensus as to the technical, economic, and scientific rationale for implementing an integrated environmental and human-health perspective with regard to workplace health and safety, there is substantial disagreement as to the legal and ethical ramifications of this perspective. Many of the key issues in current national and international dispute revolve about the issue of corporate and personal liability, especially regarding:

- The health condition of a worker that is influenced by multiple factors, only some of which are attributable to the workplace
- Workplace hazards for which there are no established standards
- Balancing the objective of minimizing workplace risk and the objective of nondiscrimination (e.g., on basis of sex, preexisting health)
- The use of medical monitoring, including genetic or other medical screening prior to and during employment
- Workplace contribution to social–environmental inequities (e.g., employing low socio-economic groups for particularly hazardous work)
- Release of naturally occurring toxic or infectious agents into a broader environment

These issues are not likely to be resolved in the near future; they will continue to influence social, legal, political, and ethical debate well into the next decade. In the meantime, a rapidly developing global economy, with its emphasis on an integration of environmental and human health management, already requires us to take a holistic view of workplace health and safety.

CHAPTER 2

HAZARD AND RISK ASSESSMENT

HAZARD AND RISK

The term *hazard* is sometimes used to define a source of potential harm or injury and, sometimes, the potential harm or injury itself. Thus, a silo containing plastic chips or grain or any other raw material may be said to be a hazard because, having entered the silo, a worker might become engulfed and subsequently asphyxiated. Or the hazard may be defined as the engulfment or the asphyxiation. This double meaning to the word hazard (i.e., the silo itself or the dangers that exist within a silo) often results in a confusion of cause and effect.

Throughout this text, the word hazard is used to denote primarily the potential harm or injury (e.g., asphyxiation) or, secondarily, the most immediate precursor to harm or injury (e.g., engulfment). This approach underscores the fact that any particular aspect of a workplace, including any single physical structure, process, procedure, as well as any single material or energy input and output may, in fact, present multiple hazards.

In this sense of the word hazard (i.e., the injury or harm itself or its most immediate precursor), a silo presents not only the hazard of asphyxiation, but also the hazard of physical injury—both of which may result from engulfment of a worker by materials stored in the silo. Moreover, asphyxiation may result not only from engulfment but, depending upon the nature of the material stored in the silo, from the lack of oxygen due to bacterial decomposition of stored organic materials or through the displacement of air by a chemical vapor. If the stored material is finely divided, explosion presents another potential hazard to both workers and the surrounding community.

Whether used in its primary or secondary sense, the word hazard always denotes a *possibility* or *potential*. This is what differentiates a hazard from a risk. Whereas a hazard is a possible (or potential) harm or injury (or an immediate precursor to harm or injury), a risk is the probability that a person will actually experience a specific hazard.

As a possibility, a hazard should be envisioned as being inherent within a substance or situation; as a probability, a risk should be envisioned as being inherent within a person's actual exposure to a substance or situation.

For example, one of the hazards of smoking cigarettes is lung cancer; this hazard is inherent in both the chemicals contained in cigarette smoke and the biochemistry of living lung cells. This is not to say that you will develop lung cancer if you smoke or that you will not develop lung cancer if you do not smoke. To say that lung cancer is a hazard associated with cigarette smoke is simply to say that cancer is a potential inherent in cigarette smoke. However, the person who inhales cigarette smoke increases his exposure to that smoke and thereby to the hazard of cancer inherent in that smoke. With increased exposure comes the increased risk of developing lung cancer (i.e., increased probability of experiencing the hazard).

The importance of distinguishing between hazard and risk (i.e., between a possibility and a probability) is that both concepts provide us with two distinct strategies for managing health and safety.

Hazard Reduction Strategy

It is often impossible to reduce a hazard. For example, one of the hazards associated with gasoline is, of course, flammability. Flammability is inherent within the chemistry of gasoline. Should it be possible to reformulate gasoline to remove this hazard, the resulting formulation would certainly not be gasoline.

However, in many instances, it is possible to reduce or effectively remove a hazard associated with a particular workplace material or process. One of the hazards of a coolant oil, for example, may be toxicity due to a heavy metal constituent (e.g., cadmium). Such an oil may easily be reformulated to remove the heavy metal constituent and thus remove the hazard of heavy metal toxicity without impairing the usefulness of the coolant. This is an example of *product reformulation*, which is an increasingly important growth industry today precisely because of the concern for human health and safety.

Another example of the hazard reduction strategy is *chemical substitution* which, though possibly involving a chemical reformulation of an existing product, primarily focuses on the substitution of a less or non-hazardous chemical or material for a more hazardous chemical or material.

Examples include water-based paint substitutes for oil-based paints, non-chlorine bleaching agents for chlorine-containing bleaching agents, and certain botanical pesticides for synthetic pesticides.

In many cases, neither chemical reformulation nor a simple chemical substitution can be directly employed. It may therefore become reasonable to consider *alternative processing engineering*, as in reengineering a water treatment plant to accomplish disinfection by an ozonation process rather than a chlorination process.

Risk Reduction Strategy

In order to reduce the risk associated with a hazard that cannot itself be reduced, it is necessary to reduce exposure. This is accomplished by implementing three *exposure-control approaches* in the following order:

a. Management control, which includes the management of schedules, assignments, and procedures and the minimization of the frequency and duration of exposure to specific hazards;
b. Engineering control, which involves the use of space, barriers, and ventilation devices to limit and isolate exposure;
c. Personal protective clothing and equipment.

Both management control and engineering control approaches are of particular importance to reducing risk not only at the workplace site, but also off-site in the surrounding community. Specific examples of management control and engineering control approaches include *efficiency improvement*, which is the redesign of production processes to improve the efficiency by which hazardous materials are processed; *in-process recycling*, which involves the rerouting of hazardous materials directly back into a production process; and *fugitive release control* (sometimes simply referred to as *housekeeping*), which includes the prevention of spills and leaks.

AGENTS AND CATEGORIES OF HAZARDS

A large diversity of physical, chemical, and biological agents can pose human health and safety hazards. Common physical agents include heat, noise, vibration, pressure, radiation, electric shock, gravitation, and cutting, abrasive, and puncturing agents. Chemical agents include tens of thousands of naturally occurring and human-made inorganic and organic chemicals. Biological agents include viruses, bacteria, and other human pathogens.

Physical, chemical, and biological agents of human hazards can be identified and described without reference to the human subjected to the associated hazard. For example, heat can burn skin, regardless of the person involved. However, there are significant hazards that are not posed by a single agent, but by the interaction of a person with his immediate environment. Such human–environment interactions are the province of *ergonomics* (also known as *human engineering* or *human factors engineering*). An example of an ergonomic source of potential hazard is the interaction of a person with a computer keyboard. Depending upon the level of the keyboard and the position of the worker's forearms, a potential hazard might be a persistent muscular spasm. Ergonomic sources of hazard are typically situations in which there is a less than ideal balance between a healthful expenditure of human energy and the energy requirements of the task being performed.

It should not be thought that the nature of the source of a hazard necessarily defines the type of hazard. For example, a chemical agent may result in a psychological hazard, such as an hallucination, or in a chemical burn. In fact, any chemical agent typically poses a variety of hazards simultaneously, including diverse physical, physiological, and psychological hazards. An ergonomically derived hazard may be a muscular, skeletal, or neurological debilitation; it may also be fatigue, or anxiety, or a host of other hazards having psychological consequence.

Table 2.1 includes a variety of hazards to be addressed in any modern programmatic approach to occupational health and safety. For convenience, hazards are categorized according to physical, chemical, and biological agents and ergonomic source. It is important to note that, while these hazards certainly pertain to the workplace environment, they are not unique to the workplace. They may be found in all aspects of contemporary life in any developed nation.

An essential aspect of any hazard assessment is the correlation of hazardous agents and sources with the immediacy and specificity of the potential harm or injury. The immediacy of a hazard is described in terms of the time interval between exposure to the hazard and the manifestation of consequent harm or injury. *Acute hazards* are those, such as corrosivity (a chemical burning of living tissue), that become manifest in a matter of seconds, hours, or a few days after exposure to the hazardous agent (e.g., sulfuric acid). *Chronic hazards* are those, such as carcinogenicity (development of a cancer), that develop only years and decades after exposure to the hazardous agent (e.g., cigarette smoke, asbestos).

The specificity of a hazard pertains to the range of its bodily affects. *Target-organ hazards* are hazards known to become manifest in specific organs or tissues (e.g., the nerves of the hand), as opposed to *systemic hazards*, which are manifest in the overall condition of the whole body (e.g., as in lead poisoning, which affects the blood, the gastrointestinal tract, and the central nervous system), or a major system of the body (e.g., as in strychnine poisoning, which acts primarily on the central nervous system).

TABLE 2.1   Examples of Hazardous Agents in the Workplace

a

Physical Agents

➤ **Acoutistic Radiation** ——— | Sonic and ultrasonic sound, including continuous and intermittent (impact) noise |

➤ **Temperature** ——— | Heat and cold stress |

➤ **Magnetic Radiation** ——— | Magnetic flux densities, including those having influence on implanted medical devices and ferromagnetic tools |

➤ **Electromagnetic Radiation** ——— | Visible light, lasers, radiofrequency/microwave radiation, ultraviolet radiation, and x-rays |

➤ **Radioactivity** ——— | Radionuclides and radiation (alpha, beta and gamma) associated with unstable atomic nuclei or nuclear reactions |

➤ **Ergonomic Stress** ——— | Stress associated with mechanical tensions in musculo-skeletal system |

➤ **Physical Impact** ——— | Mechanical impact that exerts physical force on the body |

Chemical Agents

➤ **Agents Presenting Physical Risk**

• **Asphyxiant** ——— | Vapors displace air and thereby cause suffocation |

• **Combustible** ——— | Burns when subjected to a temperature greater than 100^0F and below 200^0F |

• **Corrosive** ——— | Chemically burns living tissue on contact |

• **Explosive** ——— | Suddenly releases pressure, gas and heat when ignited |

• **Flammable** ——— | Burns when subjected to a temperature less than 100^0F |

• **Irritant** ——— | A non-corrosive material that causes itching, soreness or inflammation of exposed skin, eyes or mucous membranes |

• **Pyrophoric** ——— | Ignites spontaneously in air at temperatures of 130^0F or lower |

• **Organic Peroxide** ——— | Spontaneously explodes due to the formation of unstable peroxides |

• **Oxidizer** ——— | Promotes or initiates the burning of combustible or flammable materials |

• **Water Reactive** ——— | Reacts with water to form a flammable or toxic gas |

• **Unstable/Reactive** ——— | Spontaneously explodes with production of pressure, gas, heat and possibly toxic fumes |

continues

continued

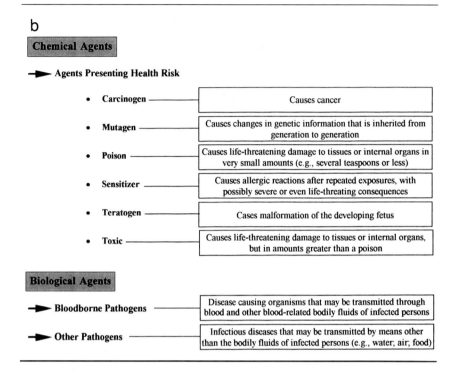

b

Chemical Agents

➤ **Agents Presenting Health Risk**

- **Carcinogen** ——— Causes cancer
- **Mutagen** ——— Causes changes in genetic information that is inherited from generation to generation
- **Poison** ——— Causes life-threatening damage to tissues or internal organs in very small amounts (e.g., several teaspoons or less)
- **Sensitizer** ——— Causes allergic reactions after repeated exposures, with possibly severe or even life-threating consequences
- **Teratogen** ——— Cases malformation of the developing fetus
- **Toxic** ——— Causes life-threatening damage to tissues or internal organs, but in amounts greater than a poison

Biological Agents

➤ **Bloodborne Pathogens** ——— Disease causing organisms that may be transmitted through blood and other blood-related bodily fluids of infected persons

➤ **Other Pathogens** ——— Infectious diseases that may be transmitted by means other than the bodily fluids of infected persons (e.g., water; air; food)

It must be stressed that the reason for differentiating between acute and chronic hazards and between target-organ and systemic hazards is not to assign priority regarding the management of hazards. Equal attention must be given to acute as well as chronic hazards and to target-organ and systemic hazards. The importance in differentiating among the immediacy and specificity of workplace hazards is, rather, to define the scope required for the effective management of health and safety hazards that characterize a particular workplace and threaten its surrounding community.

EXPOSURE: THE HOLISTIC VIEW

As the essential link between hazard (as a possibility) and risk (as a probability), exposure must be examined in detail, with specific attention given to the following dimensions:

1. Quantitative measure (such as the concentration of chemical inhaled, number of volts, wavelength of radiation, number of decibels), including not only measures of the amount or nature of the hazardous agent, but also measures of the duration and frequency of exposure
2. Pathway(s) by which the hazard comes into direct contact with human tissue (such as by inhalation, ingestion, absorption, skin, eye or bodily contact, physical penetration, sensation)
3. Mechanism(s) by which the hazard is transported or propagated from its source to a human, most often referred to as *environmental transport* or *fate*
4. Mechanism(s) by which a hazardous agent might be transformed during its transport or propagation (such as a chemical or physical transformation)
5. Individual humans or populations that might come into contact with the hazard

The quantitative measure of exposure is usually prompted by specific health and safety standards that have regulatory authority. There are, however, relatively few standards for workplace hazards. For example, there are standards for less than 1% of the total number of chemicals in daily use in a developed nation. Another reason for quantifying exposure, even in the absence of relevant standards, is the simple fact that some legal jurisdictions have established the right of the worker to know the quantitative value of his or her exposure. Finally, it is generally recognized that effective medical treatment engendered by hazardous exposure requires quantitative information about that exposure.

Where quantitative measures of exposure are made, the focus is typically on the worker; usually ignored in the day-to-day management of industrial health and safety is the exposure of, say, family members to chemical contaminants "carried" by the worker out of the workplace and into the home. Historically, quantification of such "carry home" contamination and of other community exposures to workplace hazards, such as air, water and soil contaminants, has been accomplished only in the progress of specialized community health surveys. As a more holistic, integrated approach to workplace health and safety becomes established, it can be expected that such quantification of community exposures to the hazards of individual work sites will become more common.

Today, any competent exposure analysis of industrial hazards includes a detailed description of the various specific pathways or *routes of entry* by which a hazardous agent comes into contact with living tissue. Many hazards impinge upon living tissue through different pathways. Acetone, for example, can exert a defatting effect on skin simply through physical contact; it can also be absorbed through skin tissue into the blood, inhaled into the lung, or, if an acetone mist settles onto food, ingested. The toxicity of most chemicals typically depends on the specific pathway whereby they enter the body.

Physical agents may also impinge upon the human body in different ways, depending upon various factors. Electromagnetic radiation, depending upon its wavelength, may penetrate directly through skin into deeper body layers (as with ultraviolet radiation) or be restricted essentially to the surface of the skin (as with visible light). Similarly, the energy of sound may be perceived through the ear as noise or through the body proper as a physical vibration.

The environmental transport of a hazardous agent includes all environmental pathways that the agent follows from its source to a human being; some pathways involve transformations of the agent. The term *environmental dynamics* is most often used to denote both transport and transformation processes that a particular hazardous agent may undergo after release to air, water, or soil. Generic categories of environmental dynamics include the following interactions of hazardous materials and energies with so called environmental compartments, i.e., air, water, soil, and organisms:

- *introduction* of materials and energies into major environmental compartments;
- *transformation* of materials and energies within environmental compartments;
- *translocation* of materials and energies from compartment to compartment;
- *concentration* of materials and energies within compartments;
- *dissipation* of materials and energies within compartments;
- *elimination* of materials and energies from compartments.

Figure 2.1 shows that the various environmental dynamics of a hazardous agent are highly interconnected. For example, an industrially generated contaminant such as a compound of mercury may be introduced (by improper disposal methods) into groundwater and subsequently translocated via groundwater flow to surface water where, after transformation by aquatic microorganisms, mercuric metabolites may become concentrated in fish tissue. If such fish are then harvested for human consumption, the ingested mercury may result in severe neurological damage of large numbers of humans. While the worker in the plant that generates the mercuric waste may have little if no exposure to mercury at the work-site, that same worker may suffer lethal exposure while at home. In similar fashion, a lactating female may be exposed to polybrominated biphenyls (PBBs) in her work place. Once introduced into her blood, say through inhalation, the PBBs may

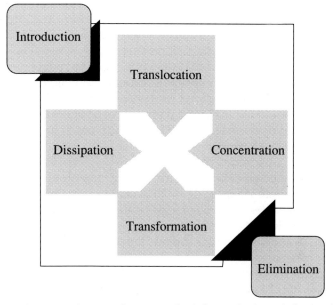

FIGURE 2.1 Generic environmental processes that influence the dynamic flows and transformations of materials and energies in environmental compartments (square) such as air, water, soil, and organisms.

concentrate in her breast milk and be subsequently introduced to her nursing infant, causing a variety of toxic effects, including death.

As these examples demonstrate, it is only through a careful examination of both the environmental transport and transformation of a hazardous agent and its route of entry that any comprehensive assessment can be made of just who may be at risk. To assume that only the on-site worker is at risk regarding workplace hazards is often to ignore precisely those who are at greatest risk.

RISK ASSESSMENT

Risk assessment is essentially an integration of the findings provided by a hazard assessment and an exposure assessment; it is the basis for formulating health and safety policy and for implementing a strategy of prevention. Today, risk assessment takes many forms and is inclusive of diverse objectives and techniques.

When carried out by a governmental agency, risk assessment is typically the prelude to establishing regulatory or advisory (i.e., legally non-mandatory) health and safety standards. When performed by an insurance company, the purpose is to establish premium rates or to advise corporate clients as to corrective actions that should be taken to reduce financial and legal risks associated with workplace health and safety. When performed by a professional association such as, in the United States, the National Fire Prevention Association (NFPA), the purpose is to promote the most prudent guidelines regarding the management of specific types of hazards. These are typically matters well beyond the immediate authority of the health and safety officer of a particular company who, though benefiting greatly from the information and guidance provided by these organizations and authorities, has no practical influence on or contribution to such information and guidance. Nonetheless, when conducted by the in-plant safety officer, a risk assessment is nothing less than the factual basis for formulating a workplace-specific health and safety policy and for implementing a workplace-specific strategy of prevention.

Perhaps the elements of a written risk assessment can be most easily defined in terms of a multi- or n-dimensional matrix: along one axis, headings reflect the totality of operations, energetic and material inputs, products, and by-products that characterize a specific plant; along other axes, major headings reflect information regarding the hazard and exposure assessments conducted for that plant. As already discussed, this information includes (for each identified operation, input, product, and by-product) a specific hazardous agent or source, acute and chronic effects, target-organ and systemic effects, key environmental dynamics and consequent routes of entry, on- and off-site persons likely to be exposed, alternative hazard reduction strategies, and (ultimately) alternative risk reduction strategies.

Other categorical types of information essential to a risk assessment and which must be integrated into such an n-dimensional matrix include *risk factors* (i.e., personal attributes that place specific groups of persons at high risk) and *equity factors* (i.e., demographic criteria that are useful for describing the social distribution of risks).

Risk factors of particular importance include (a) general health conditions of persons that are typically non-job-related but which can be exacerbated by their employment (e.g., preexisting heart condition, allergy, high blood pressure), (b) genetic propensity toward certain health problems (e.g., multiple sclerosis, leukemia), (c) behavior (e.g., smoking, alcoholism, abuse of controlled substances), (d) reproductive state (e.g., sensitivity of developing fetus to teratogens and other toxic substances, mutagenic and toxic effects on human ova and sperm), and (e) gender-enhanced susceptibility to accumulation and/or effects of toxins (e.g., longer retention time of benzene in females, enhanced sensitivity to lead-induced changes in red blood cells in

females, enhanced susceptibility to dimethylbenazanthracene-induced geno-
toxicity in males).

Largely ignored throughout the past several decades of the environmental movement, the issue of social equity (sometimes called *environmental
equity*) is of increasing concern. Certainly in the contemporary holistic approach to environmental and human interactions, the manner in which environmental risks (including occupationally related health and safety risks)
are socially distributed is not only of national but also of international social,
economic, and political interest.

In describing populations at specific risk due to workplace attributes
and operations, it is therefore, if not legally required, at least instructive to
consider whether or not such risks are equitably distributed with regard to
such demographic factors as gender, race, ethnicity, age, and socio-economic
class. Depending upon historical and cultural aspects of a particular nation,
it may be necessary to consider additional factors (e.g., religious affiliation,
level of formal education, geographic location).

There is no question that the inclusion of any consideration of personal risk factors and societywide equity factors in the analysis of occupationally related health and safety raises particularly sensitive issues of legal,
ethical, and sociological import. However, the very purpose of a formal risk
assessment process is to predicate a policy of risk management on a comprehensive understanding of "real" risks. What in fact constitutes a "real" risk
is not determined simply by physical, chemical, or biological parameters but
also by social perceptions and political sensitivities. The workplace and what
happens there (and elsewhere because of it) are no longer within the private
province of the owner or even of the state or nation in which it is located.

CHAPTER 3

OCCUPATIONAL HEALTH AND SAFETY STANDARDS

ACCEPTABLE RISK

In the day-to-day management of workplace health and safety, a standard is typically used as a practical measure of regulatory compliance. Should the workplace meet applicable standards, the likely conclusion might understandably be that the workplace is safe—that the health and safety of workers is assured.

The widespread preoccupation with regulatory compliance with health and safety standards and the consubstantiation of "meeting standards" and "working safely," while understandable, can nonetheless mislead a safety officer into a false sense of security, most commonly because of a basic misunderstanding of certain statistical concepts that underlie any standard, or of the technical meaning of the word "safe," or of the scientific and normative procedures used in the process of setting standards.

In essence, any standard is a judgment as to what constitutes a *socially acceptable risk*. As discussed in Chapter 2, a health or safety risk is always a probability. Therefore a standard is a judgment as to what specific probability of harm or injury is to be considered socially acceptable. While it would certainly be desirable to define an acceptable risk as "zero," this is not possible. A zero probability implies omniscience—an absolute guarantee that something will not happen—which is not a scientifically acceptable assumption. Any socially acceptable risk is therefore always greater than zero. In short, to equate "compliance with a standard" with "achieving a safe condition" is simply to say that, by complying with a standard we assume that actual health and safety incidents will be within socially acceptable limits—

not that such incidents will not occur but, rather, that they will occur at such a low frequency that society as a whole will not deem corrective action necessary.

Consider, for example, a hypothetical situation in which a certain toxic contaminant in a drinking water supply presents the risk of one person out of a total population of one million suffering brain damage. The risk of brain damage is therefore one in a million (1/1,000,000, or 10^{-7}). Imagine also that, should the concentration of this contaminant increase, the risk will increase—say to one in one hundred thousand, to one in ten thousand, and even, ultimately, to one in ten. Obviously, somewhere along this range of risks from 10^{-7} to 10^{-1}, which is, after all, the difference between one person in a very large city and one person in our immediate family suffering brain damage, the risk becomes personal. Where we draw the line—that point along the range of probabilities at which we decide the risk is no longer acceptable—is analogous to setting a standard. Of course, occupational health and safety standards, as well as environmental quality standards, are not set on the basis of our personal levels of tolerance of risk. They are intended to reflect a collective tolerance, a social acceptability of risk.

Because standards depend upon an assessment of just what is socially acceptable and what is not, it is necessary to emphasize that standards, although they are based on highly technical and scientific considerations, are essentially judgments and are therefore subject to the common limitations of any human judgment.

One particular limitation regarding health and safety standards derives simply from the fact that a standard is a judgment of the social acceptability of risk. For example, in the United States, a commonly used measure of the social acceptability of risk regarding carcinogenic chemicals (i.e., chemicals that can cause cancer) is 10^{-7}. This means that an exposure of a million persons to a carcinogen that results in a single occurrence of cancer *in excess of what would occur without such an exposure* is considered beyond social acceptability (i.e., the exposure exceeds the standard).

There is no scientific necessity for setting the acceptable risk of carcinogenicity at 10^{-7}; those who promulgate this very risk argue that it reflects the long entrenched fear of cancer in American society. The argument is strengthened by contemporary national statistics that show cancer accounting for roughly 20+% of deaths due to known causes and also by the common observation that Americans are much less tolerant of risks that they do not know or understand and over which they exercise little or no control than those they do understand and over which they may exercise at least some control (e.g., safety risks associated with motor vehicles).

International Context

The American experience is not necessarily, of course, the experience of the rest of the world. In a nation in which death may be due primarily to infectious disease or even starvation, a much higher risk of carcinogenicity might well be socially acceptable and a correspondingly higher exposure standard more practicably relevant. The broad implementation of any particular health and safety standard in the international context of diverse social realities therefore raises profoundly complex social, political, economic, and ethical issues, especially in a period of enhanced global sensitivity to social and cultural pluralism.

Not only might the relevance of a particular standard depend upon diverse national and cultural definitions of social acceptability, but also upon key technical variables that influence human health profiles. In this regard, it is essential to emphasize that human health is always a multidimensional phenomenon. While such factors of general nutrition, the quality of drinking water, housing, education, and family income are of broad demographic, social, and political interest, they are also integral variables in the health profile of any human population. Workers derived from different populations who, because of such variables, likely bring different general health profiles into the workplace, may reasonably be expected to experience different levels of workplace protection while working even under the same occupational standard.

Environmental Equity

The potential disparity in protection engendered by the rigorously equal application of a health standard to populations having unequal health profiles is not simply of interest to the international community, but also within individual nations.

In the United States , there is increasing concern that there may be a significantly disproportionate distribution of health risks among racial and ethnic minorities due to such key environmental attributes as air and water quality. In response to this concern for what is commonly referred to as "environmental justice" or "environmental equity," the President issued Executive Order 12898 (February 11, 1994), which requires each Federal agency to ". . . make achieving environmental justice part of its mission by identifying and addressing, as appropriate, disproportionately high and adverse human health or environmental effects of its programs, policies, and activities on minority populations and low-income populations in the United States . . ." Environmental inequities addressed in this Executive Order could well result, if not resolved, in an enhanced occupational risk for minority as compared to majority populations working at the same workplace and under the same health standards.

Jurisdiction and Legal Standing

Finally, irrespective of the influence of either diverse cultural definitions of "acceptable risk" or the potential effect of the environment on human health, or even social inequities regarding the general health profiles of prospective workers, the legal standing of the normative process used in setting standards is itself a source of concern over the relevance and the efficacy of any particular workplace standard.

In some instances, legal jurisdictions regarding the setting of standards are confused by the sheer multiplicity of governmental agencies having diverse authorities, the relative role of legislative, executive, and judicial functions, and the proliferation of professional organizations.

In the United States, for example, the Federal Occupational Safety and Health Administration (OSHA) has the prime responsibility for establishing and promulgating workplace safety and health standards for workers involved in interstate commerce. The authority of the Federal OSHA *vis-à-vis* State OSHAs is continually subject to litigation regarding not only variable legal interpretations of just what constitutes interstate commerce, but also administrative constraints imposed by Congress on the Federal OSHA with regard to specific procedures followed in adopting specific standards— constraints that have precluded the Federal OSHA from adopting workplace standards recommended by the American Conference of Governmental Industrial Hygienists (ACGIH), which (despite the implication of its name) is not a governmental agency.

Federal and state common law regarding tort liability in the United States also reflects a diversity of interpretations regarding the legal status of a workplace health and safety standard. Some courts have determined that a company's violation of a statutory health and safety standard that is directly related to the type of harm actually suffered by a plaintiff worker conclusively establishes tort liability for that company; other courts have held that such a violation of an OSHA standard is merely evidence of possible negligence that the jury must consider along with other evidence. While courts have typically determined that a company's compliance (or noncompliance) with an OSHA standard should at least be considered as some measure of the company's reasonable care for the health and safety of a worker, courts have also emphasized that a statutory standard should be considered a minimum goal. However, it has also been suggested in the juridical literature that a statutory standard may in fact be less protective of the worker than what a jury may ultimately decide should be a company's reasonable care and concern for its workers' health and safety.

Influence of Global Economy

Traditionally, and despite the variability inherent in the political pluralism of individual societies, health and safety standards have been essentially the province of the nation. However, with the advent of a global economy and its consequent emphasis on an integrated paradigm of environmental quality and human health, national standards can be expected to become increasingly influenced by the realities of international business. Perhaps of particular relevance is the growing body of international manufacturing standards that encompass not only concern for quality assurance of products and services, but also for the impact of industrial processes and products on environmental quality and human health.

The broad goal of the International Standards Organization (ISO) is "to promote the development of standardization and related activities in the world with a view to facilitating international exchange of goods and services, and to develop cooperation in the sphere of intellectual, scientific, technological and economic activity." A key objective in attaining this goal was achieved by the establishment (in 1987) of a set of quality standards generally known as the ISO 9000 series. These standards encompass (a) a certification procedure for companies involved in international commerce, (b) standards for the production, installation, and servicing of products, (c) facility inspection and product testing, and (d) quality assurance certification. While these standards are very general and, to date, minimally prescriptive regarding workplace operations, they are specifically intended to establish a certification procedure that is applicable to a continually expanding number of companies and which will progressively prescribe international environmental quality criteria.

In essence, the clear intent of ISO is to provision a company's entry into international trade on the basis of a facility audit, external confirmation of broad compliance with environmental quality and human health standards, and the public disclosure of managerial failings.

Typically known within the international community as the *harmonizing of international environmental quality criteria*, this objective can be expected to provide a major impetus to the examination and reevaluation of traditional paradigms that underlie conventional business, legal institutions, and contemporary national approaches to the management of health, safety, and the environment (HSE). Already there is significant international movement to consider HSE an integral component of *Total Quality Management*; to reexamine the constraints imposed upon the English common law (and its diverse, global legal progeny) by now historically dated agricultural and early industrial preoccupation with questions of property, possession, and fault; to recast the goal of short-term profit to one of long-term sustainability; and to accomplish the wholesale expansion of the public's right to access to all information that impacts human health. It cannot be expected that, in light of such considerations, either the substance or the philosophy of the occupational safety and health standards of any individual nation will long remain unaffected.

Data Base for Standards

A safety and health standard regarding a particular hazard may be based on historical experience with the hazard (usually in the workplace), laboratory studies (of animals and, to a much lesser extent, humans), and epidemiological studies (statistical studies of large numbers of people). Each of these approaches has its unique advantages and disadvantages, and each must be considered in any comprehensive review of the health effects of any hazardous agent. An excellent example of such comprehensive reviews of toxic chemicals is the series of toxicological profiles published by the U.S. Agency for Toxic Substances and Disease Registry (Public Health Service; U.S. Department of Health and Human Services; Washington, DC).

Historical experience is often in the form of reported case studies of health or safety incidents as, for example, in studies of workers exposed to styrene vapors in the production of plastics and polystyrene resins. By themselves, case studies of particular incidents are often of very limited value because of imprecise quantitative measures of actual exposure to the hazardous agent (e.g., a range of styrene concentrations as opposed to specific values), minimal data regarding the health history of persons involved in a particular incident, and, typically, the relatively small number of people affected.

Laboratory studies provide essential data on the relationship between quantitative exposure to a hazardous agent (e.g., how much and for how long) and the effect of exposure (e.g., lethality, reproductive toxicity). This relationship, expressed as a *dose–response curve* (Figure 3.1), is the ultimate basis of any standard. However, dose–response curves based on laboratory studies of animals are subject to much ongoing scientific debate regarding their relevance to human health, especially regarding the relatively large doses utilized in such experiments (both in terms of amounts of the hazardous agent and the frequency and duration of exposure). Despite the former extensive use of volunteers, prisoners, and even unknowing or purposely mislead military personnel, institutionalized children, and other citizens, laboratory experiments involving human exposure to hazardous agents are

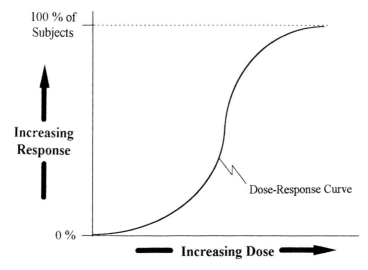

FIGURE 3.1   The dose–response curve, which correlates an increasing probability (risk) of experiencing a toxic response with an increasing dose of toxic chemical.

today necessarily narrowly prescribed by law. Limited essentially to highly specialized trials of therapeutic pharmaceuticals, laboratory experiments are therefore of negligible value regarding the process of setting occupational standards.

An epidemiological study of a hazardous agent focuses directly on humans. The key objective, as with a laboratory study, is to establish a dose–response curve. However, while the researcher absolutely controls actual dose in a laboratory study, the researcher cannot control dose in an epidemiological study. Rather, the exposures of persons included in an epidemiological study of a hazardous agent are determined experientially—by their work, their home life, their general life-style. In some instances, subjects expose themselves willingly, as do those who smoke cigarettes; in others, subjects are exposed unknowingly (e.g., residents in homes containing radon gas) or unwillingly (e.g., nonsmokers who breathe in "second-hand" smoke).

The Dose–Response Curve

Figure 3.2 depicts an example of the relationship between the dose of a toxic chemical expressed as weight of the chemical (mg) per unit of body weight (kg) and the effect (e.g., lethality) of that chemical. As shown in the figure, the sigmoid dose–response curve is the mathematical integral (i.e.,

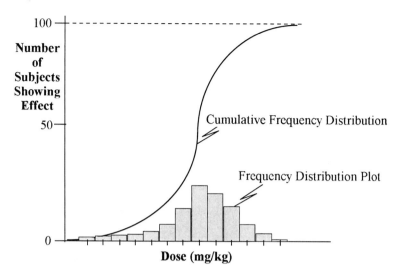

FIGURE 3.2   The dose–response curve is often referred to as the integral of a frequency distribution plot because it represents the cumulative effect of an increasing dose of toxic chemical.

cumulative total) of the frequency distribution plot (often called the quantal response plot or curve). The frequency distribution plot reflects the fact that any biological population is composed of individuals who have different physiological sensitivities to the same dose of a toxic chemical, with some being relatively sensitive, and others, relatively tolerant. The integral of the frequency distribution plot (i.e., the sigmoid dose–response curve) encompasses the total population of individuals, and is therefore inclusive of the full range of variable sensitivities within the subject population.

While the vertical ordinate of the sigmoid dose–response curve (hereafter called the dr–curve) denotes the percentage (of the total population) demonstrating the lethal effect of a particular dose of toxic chemical, that percentage can be interpreted as a probability (i.e., risk). Thus, 20% can be interpreted as a 2-out-of-10 (or 0.2) risk. This means that, for every 10 persons receiving a particular dose, two can be expected to die—if a single person receives that same dose, the probability (or risk) of death is still 2 out of 10.

Information about the toxicity of a chemical that is typically available to a safety officer includes the dose of that chemical that will result in a 5-out-of-10 risk (or 0.5 probability) of death. This dose is referred to as the LD_{50}, or lethal dose for 50% of the population receiving that dose. This statistic essentially states that any one subject exposed to the LD_{50} has a 0.5

TABLE 3.1   Relative Toxicity of Chemicals on the Basis of LD$_{50}$ Values

Relative toxicity	LD$_{50}$ (mg/kg)[a]	Lethal amount[b]	Examples of chemicals[c]
Extremely toxic (poison)	<1	<7 drops	Dioxin Botulinus toxin Tetrodotoxin
Highly toxic (poison)	1–50	7 drops–1 teaspoon	Hydrogen cyanide Nickel oxide Arsenic trioxide
Very toxic	50–500	1 teaspoon–1 ounce	Methylene chloride Phenol DDT
Moderately toxic	500–5000	1 ounce–1 pint	Benzene Chloroform Chromium chloride
Slightly toxic	>5000	>1 pint	Acetone Ethyl alcohol Ferrous sulfate

[a] As tested by the oral route in rats.
[b] Lethal amount for average adult human, based on liquid with density of water.
[c] As tested by various routes in several animal species.

probability of dying. If some toxic effect of exposure other than lethality is denoted (e.g., loss of hair, impaired learning), the equivalent statistic is expressed as ED$_{50}$, for "effective dose."

Where LD$_{50}$ or ED$_{50}$ are used, dose strictly implies the amount of chemical actually taken into the body of the subject organism. In some instances, toxicity information is presented in terms of LC$_{50}$ or EC$_{50}$, which refer, respectively, to lethal and effective concentrations of the toxic chemical in the ambient atmosphere or water.

Values of LD$_{50}$ or LC$_{50}$ are useful for describing relative toxicities. For example, Table 3.1 includes LD$_{50}$ values and commonly used categories of relative toxicity. Although these terms are in general use, LD$_{50}$ values do have important limitations with respect to comparing the toxicity of two or more chemicals. Figure 3.3 depicts the straight line portions of the dr–curves for two different chemicals. Although both chemicals have equal LD$_{50}$s, increasing the dose of one chemical results in a smaller incremental increase in risk than does increasing the dose of the other. The safety officer is therefore well advised to be wary about describing the relative toxicity of workplace chemicals solely in terms of LD$_{50}$ values.

The dr–curve of a hazardous agent can provide extremely important information regarding the lowest dose at which an adverse health effect can be expected. For example, Figure 3.4 depicts the dr–curves for two chemicals.

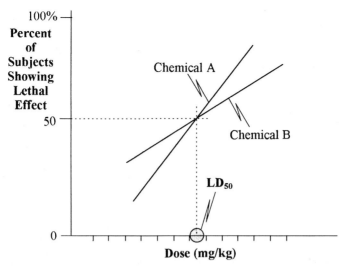

FIGURE 3.3   The straight-line portions of two dose–response curves for two different chemicals having the same LD_{50}. Note that, at doses less than the LD_{50}, chemical A is less toxic than chemical B, whereas the opposite is true at higher doses. This illustrates the fallacy of trying to use LD_{50} values to describe the relative toxicities of two or more chemicals.

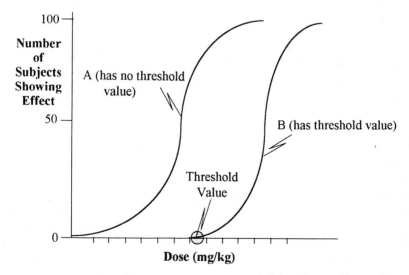

FIGURE 3.4   Some chemicals (A) cause an increasing probability of toxic effects with every incremental increase in dose; others (B) may cause no toxic effects until the dose reaches a threshold value. Whether or not a chemical has a threshold value above "zero" can only be determined by experiment.

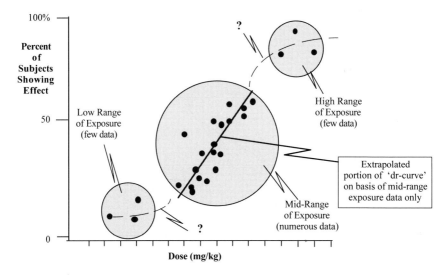

FIGURE 3.5 Epidemiological data (black circles) tend to be least numerous at low and high ranges of exposure to a toxic chemical and most numerous at the mid-range. Mathematical extrapolations of data points are therefore poor at low and high ranges of exposure (dotted lines), and most reliable within the mid-range of exposure (solid line). This means that epidemiological data are typically not useful for determining whether a chemical has a low-range threshold value.

One of the curves shows a *threshold value*, which is a dose below which no adverse health effect is observed; the other shows a probability of adverse health effect for every dose greater than zero—it has no threshold value.

It is important to consider that the presence or absence of a threshold value for a particular hazardous agent can be defined only with respect to a particular type of effect. For example, a known threshold decibel value with regard to "significant loss of hearing" (which is reflected in a noise standard) is totally irrelevant with respect to another type of health effect of noise, such as "irritability" (which is not reflected in a noise standard).

Another important consideration regarding threshold values is that they usually cannot be detected by means of epidemiological studies. As shown in Figure 3.5, epidemiological studies typically generate few data at the extreme ranges of human exposures to hazardous agents. Few extremely high exposures are included simply because relatively few people experience extremely high doses; few extremely low doses are included simply because, at such low doses, there is little if any cause either to measure or to document such exposures. At both extremes, then, the dr–curve must be extrapolated from the mid-range of more frequently observed exposures—a procedure that, despite its mathematical elegance, does not document what actually happens at either extreme and certainly, at low exposures, cannot detect a threshold.

SCIENTIFIC BIAS

While it is generally agreed that epidemiological studies generate the type of data most directly relevant to occupational exposures, such studies also include (as does any study) inherent biases that can limit their usefulness for setting workplace standards.

Among the many requisites of a well designed epidemiological study, a large subject population and one exposed to a hazardous agent over a long period of time are key requirements. A large population is needed in order to define the statistical significance of the study's findings; a long period of exposure is required to allow for the development of chronic effects in the subject population.

With regard to an epidemiological study of workplace exposure, the likelihood is, therefore, that the subject population will be male, because it is only in recent years that females have become a large portion of the out-of-home industrial work force and, even now, only in some industries. The second likelihood is that the males who constitute the subject population will have begun their employment when they were relatively young—there is no other way of ensuring a long-term exposure. The third likelihood is that these males, who began to work (and therefore began their workplace exposure to hazardous agents) when they were young, will by and large have lived basically healthy lives throughout the period covered by the study as a consequence of their having survived a long work-life.

Most frequently called the "young, healthy male syndrome" of epidemiological studies of the industrial workplace, these likely characteristics of the subject population necessarily mean that the findings of such studies necessarily reflect what happens to young, healthy males. Because studies methodologically biased in this manner influence the setting of workplace standards, it may be said that the resultant standards apply essentially to young healthy males—certainly not to females, regardless of their general health, and not to males who are neither young nor healthy.

The long known young, healthy male syndrome of epidemiological studies of the workplace exists simply because, historically, it has been young, healthy males who have had most of the consistent workplace experience in technologically developed societies. However, this broadly acknowledged source of methodological bias is also compounded by other factors that influence the data base open to epidemiological query and which are charged with a wide range of social and political emotions and sensitivities—namely, the degree to which any historically defined work force reflects racial and ethnic inequities in the access of people both to certain types of industry and, within any particular industry, to different types of jobs (and, therefore, of exposures). Certainly in this period of nascent globalization of national economies it is incumbent upon us to consider how the demographics of racism as well as of sexism have skewed even our most sophisticated scientific understanding of how hazardous agents in the workplace may in fact affect humans—not just the socially selected (or deselected) few, but the collective all.

Another type of bias that influences our scientific understanding of hazardous workplace agents emanates not from the population considered, but from the type of health effects considered. Sometimes the type of health effects considered depends upon factors only remotely related to concerns for occupational safety and health.

For example, one of the hallmarks of any scientific study is its replicatibility—its capacity to yield consistently comparable results when performed by other investigators. For the scientist, this requirement enforces the objective definition of any measurements to be performed, including the measurement of the response side of the dose–response equation. The proliferation of LD_{50} values in the scientific literature available to the safety officer attests to the fact that lethality is perhaps the most objective measure of toxicological response. Few researchers, after all, will disagree as to which experimental animals are dead or alive. Yet the modern management of health and safety in the workplace requires managerial attention to the full range of possible effects of hazardous agents—a range that includes but is not limited to lethality. While currently available workplace health and safety standards attempt to address the multiplicity of effects associated with exposure to workplace hazards, it is clear that there is much disparity in the amount of scientific effort devoted to the elucidation of different effects.

THRESHOLD LIMIT VALUES

Occupational health and safety standards for atmospheric concentrations of hazardous substances are expressed in terms of *threshold limit values*, which represent either concentrations of chemicals or measurements of physical agents (noise, heat, radiation, etc.) under which it is presumed that the vast majority of persons may perform their daily work without adverse effects. Some standards regarding chemical exposures are expressed as *biological exposure indices*, which are considered as reference values for evaluating potential health hazards. The key difference between threshold limit values (TLVs) and biological exposure indices (BEIs) is that the former apply to the ambient workplace while the latter apply to the actual tissues or bodily fluids of the worker. TLVs should therefore be viewed as essentially proactive standards because they can be used to manage risks prior to actual insults to the health and safety of the worker. While BEIs do not necessarily indicate an actual health risk, measurements of bodily specimens that persistently exceed BEIs do indicate the need for corrective action; BEIs should therefore be viewed as essentially reactive standards.

As the primary proactive means of monitoring the efficacy of health and safety management practices in the workplace, a TLV may be represented by different types of values:

1. Time weighted average (TWA) for an 8-hr work day and a 40-hr work week,
2. Short-term exposure limit (STEL), which is usually a 15-min TWA exposure limit, and/or
3. Ceiling (C), a value that should not be exceeded for any period of time.

As an average, a TWA, which is by far the most commonly available of the three types of TLV, permits exposures greater than the indicated standard for various periods of the work day as long as there are compensatory periods of reduced exposure. Regulatory agencies that promulgate TWAs provide detailed guidelines regarding limits imposed on periodic increases above TWAs (so-called *excursion limits*) that may be compensated by periods of reduced exposure. Neither STEL nor C values may be compensated for by any period of reduced exposure; they should be considered as absolute constraints on exposure to substances that present particularly acute risks to the worker.

It is important that the safety officer understand that a threshold limit value standard, whether expressed as a TWA, STEL, or C, is not identical to a toxicological threshold value as discussed above with reference to a dr–curve. The toxicological threshold value, which is frequently called the *biological threshold*, is a dose below which no adverse biological response is observed in a laboratory controlled or epidemiologically based scientific study. A TLV is a dose below which no adverse health effects are expected to occur among nearly all exposed workers. The former concept of "threshold" is a scientifically derived datum; the latter concept of threshold is a normatively derived judgment that is informed by scientific knowledge but which must also take account of broader human experience.

Perceptions of Standards

Because standards are typically expressed quantitatively and, as in the case of time weighted averages, subject to universally accepted mathematical algorithms, because they incorporate essentially consensual scientific knowledge, and because they are typically promulgated in the name of legal authority, health and safety standards are all too often viewed as absolute guarantees as opposed to normative judgments. The professional industrial hygienist and other human health practitioners know better—that workplace health and safety standards are most appropriately viewed as absolute but minimal requirements for managing the health and safety of workers. However, the management of workplace health and safety in the vast majority of workplaces throughout the world, including the more than six million company sites in the United States, is not in the hands of the professionally trained industrial hygienist or other human health professional.

The typical safety officer is a manager, production worker, or regulatory compliance officer who, having been assigned health and safety responsibility, derives relevant training from on-the-job experience with health and safety matters and from periodic, short-term training courses and workshops offered primarily by the private sector service industry and, secondarily, by regulatory authorities. In the United States, the responsibility for in-plant health and safety is increasingly given to the human resource manager or to the plant operations manager, but production personnel having part-time health and safety responsibilities continue to fulfill the role of safety officer in the vast majority of companies.

Recognizing the need for a more professional training of the typical corporate safety officer, colleges and universities have begun to expand both undergraduate and graduate training in occupational health and safety, with particular emphasis on the integration of health and safety with business management curricula. Despite these recent developments, the typical corporate safety officer has little if any formal education in industrial hygiene or the human health professions and, pressed by regulatory agencies, who are intent on regulatory compliance, and by upper corporate management, which is intent on maximizing the efficiency of production while minimizing legal liability, continues to perceive compliance with occupational health and safety standards as the sole objective. This perception must be clearly understood to contravene the following principles regarding the proper meaning and use of health and safety standards:

1. No standard can be used as a fine distinction between what is safe and what is dangerous or between so-called relative degrees of safety and danger. As judgments, standards are recommendations; while they are based on the best information available, standards are still recommendations and imply no guarantee whatsoever.

2. Compliance with a legally enforceable health and safety standard does not necessarily imply absolution from legal liability. While there is much diversity among the world's legal systems, it is quite commonly held that

personal responsibility does not stop at the point of regulatory compliance. Nor should it be overlooked that legal responsibility generally does not define the limits of moral or ethical responsibility.

3. No health or safety standard is intended in any way to invalidate or confute the premise that the best practice is always to minimize human contact with hazardous agents.

4. As judgments based on human experience, health and safety standards are changeful—they reflect not only changes in our knowledge and understanding, but also changes in our technology (e.g., the techniques for measuring concentrations of contaminants) and in social values and expectations.

5. No health or safety standard should be used in the absence of a detailed understanding of all technical and scientific aspects of the standard, including requirements related to ambient and personal monitoring, data handling and management, and quality control.

6. The absence of a standard does not in any way imply that a hazard does not exist or that no action should be taken to manage a worker's potential risk.

CHAPTER 4

THE HSE AUDIT

FACILITY AUDITS: AN OVERVIEW

Over the past two decades, companies have discovered the usefulness of the facility audit as a basic tool for managing their performance regarding environmental quality and occupational health and safety. Sometimes, facility audits focus narrowly on a particular issue, such as compliance with specific regulations (e.g., hazardous waste regulations, process safety regulations, etc.), a particular type of certification (e.g., certification under the International Standards Organization [ISO]), and the specific requirements of contractual or economic instruments (e.g., insurance policies, mortgages, and loans, etc.). Sometimes the purpose for conducting a facility audit is much more broad, such as prioritizing objectives over a wide range of environmental and health and safety issues, preparing for comprehensive plant inspections by governmental or even high level corporate managers, and enhancing the image of the plant as projected to both its employees and the general public.

Depending upon the purpose of the audit and a variety of other factors, including costs, availability of personnel, the sensitivity of the issue being examined, and legal ramifications, facility audits are commonly conducted by (a) corporate personnel, (b) external professional consultants, (c) selected local authorities, and/or (d) professional or *ad hoc* associations.

Audits performed by corporate personnel offer the obvious advantages of low cost and privacy. Whether conducted by a single person, such as a facility manager, an on-site safety officer or compliance officer, or by a team, which may include off-site corporate personnel as well as on-site managerial and production personnel, in-house audits are generally conducted at a higher frequency than are audits performed by "outsiders." Today, many plant managers even require weekly audits. While it is often thought that in-house audits are most desirable because they are conducted by persons having intimate knowledge of plant layout and operations, it is also well recognized that such intimacy can actually detract from the objectivity of an audit. The loss of objectivity is most often manifested in the oversight or casual disregard of possible problems simply because potential structural or operational causes of those problems conform to what is considered as being normal for that plant. Also, social relationships among plant personnel as well as concerns for job security may preclude a thorough investigation of actual plant conditions.

External consultants are often used precisely because they are expected to be able to exercise a fresh and objective judgment regarding plant layout and operations. Moreover, they can be selected on the basis of the particular relevance of their specialized experience and knowledge for the purpose of the audit. The high costs and sometimes prolonged effort of in-house personnel associated with selecting and using a competent consulting plant auditor typically result in a low frequency of plant audits. Also, given growing corporate concern for potential liability, many companies have found it prudent to contract a consultant only through company legal counsel in the attempt to erect the "lawyer–client privilege" between the consultant and an external authority having access to the power of subpoena. The legal efficacy of this strategy is sufficiently unclear as to sometimes preclude the use of a consultant in a situation deemed by the company to be particularly sensitive with regard to the public or governmental agencies.

In the United States, governmental agencies having responsibility for environmental quality and occupational health and safety have, in recent years, come under increasing political pressure to expand their public image of simply "enforcers" to include also "collaborator"—to become a provider not only of punishment but also of assistance. Toward this end, city, state, and federal agencies have begun to expend significant effort to work with companies proactively, an approach that has long been the hallmark of local fire departments. There is still, of course, good reason for any company to be concerned as to the wisdom of inviting regulatory agencies into its facility to conduct or participate in a facility audit that may, in fact, devolve into a "shopping spree" for regulatory infractions. There is also good reason for any regulatory agency, which is typically highly constrained in terms of budget and field personnel, to refuse to provide what are essentially free consulting services to private industry, or what may be construed by the company as an agency's "seal-of-approval," which might have relevance to subsequent legal proceedings. Despite these very real concerns and complex issues, any company that is determined to make a good-faith effort toward compliance with environmental and human health objectives is well advised at least to consider using regulatory personnel in the conduct of a facility audit.

A second discernible trend in recent years, at both the national and the international level, is the use of professional or *ad hoc* associations in both the design and the conduct of a plant audit. An appropriate professional association might be, for example, a regional association of electroplaters, a local association of metal working industries, or a national or even international association of labor. In some instances, an *ad hoc* association of particular industries and governmental agencies may be available, such as one expressly constituted to facilitate the adaptation of pollution control devices or procedures used in large manufacturing plants to small plants. In many instances, such associations include representatives of not only a particular industry (e.g., furniture manufacturing), but also the vendors of that industry (e.g., paint and varnish suppliers). The broad experience represented by such associations can be of inestimable value in both formulating and conducting an in-plant audit. Of course, any company considering such an approach must satisfy itself that it will not open the doors of its facility only to provide an advantage to business competitors.

Regardless of its specific purpose or the particular persons who conduct it, a typical facility audit undertaken to meet environmental or health and safety objectives today includes consideration of at least (a) physical structures and plant layout, (b) stock materials and wastes, (c) operational procedures, (d) personnel, and (e) records. The basic approach is to identify how these site-specific elements may individually or in combination result in or contribute to or otherwise exacerbate the air, water, soil, or organism-mediated presentation of risks to environmental quality and/or human health.

Depending upon the scope of the audit, specific elements are given more or less attention. For example, if the primary purpose of the audit is to ensure compliance with hazardous waste regulations, only those substances legally defined as hazardous wastes will likely be considered, as will only those structures, operations, personnel, and records that pertain to the management of hazardous wastes. If the purpose is to ensure compliance with so-called "chemical process safety" regulations (which owe their relatively recent genesis to the disaster in Bhopal), only those toxic substances identified in the pertinent regulations will be governing. Obviously, if the purpose of the audit is sufficiently broad—for example, to determine potential corporate legal and financial liability or even potential criminal liability—there is a much greater likelihood that all site-specific elements will be given comparable and highly detailed attention.

Without denigrating the importance of a facility audit as a useful tool for achieving a range of narrowly defined objectives, it is necessary to emphasize that the contemporary integrated approach to environmental quality and human health and safety requires the broadest possible approach to the audit process. In fact, in view of the paltry historical attention given to either environmental quality or human health and safety throughout the greater part of the industrial revolution, it is finally time to stress that, in accordance with recent litigation in the United States and elsewhere, the breadth and depth of a workplace audit should precisely reflect the deep concern that corporate owners, managers, and supervisors should have for their personal potential liability under both criminal and civil law.

HSE PERSPECTIVE

The integration of human health and safety with environmental quality objectives (HSE) under the integrated Environmental Planning and Management paradigm (Chapter 1) is predicated not only on a common appreciation of economic efficiency, but also on the growing cognizance of the essential artificiality of any clear demarcation between workplace and non-workplace experience. Just as chemical contaminants recognize no political boundary between states or nations, neither environmental nor human health determinants or consequences wholly begin or wholly end at the perimeter of the workplace. The workplace is, after all, but one dimension of the multidimensional continuum of human health and environmental quality.

This holistic HSE approach to occupational health and safety requires a more comprehensive identification of workplace attributes than has been traditionally used in the conduct of a typical facility audit. The following examples demonstrate this need:

Example 4.1 Laboratory technicians complain about a high frequency of headaches and mild nausea. After a thorough examination of potential causes, the source of the problem is determined to be exhausts from trucks that serve a food distribution warehouse in the immediate vicinity; on calm days, these exhausts often become entrained in the laboratory's ventilation system.

- *Item:* Did the plant audit focus on only the company's property?
- *Item:* How was the placement of the company's air intakes determined— was it left to the ventilator contractor to decide on the basis simply of costs and standard practice? Was any consideration given to the environs of the plant?
- *Item:* In identifying potential chemical risks for plant personnel, did the safety officer focus only on chemicals used at or produced by the company?

Example 4.2 After extensive new landscaping of its headquarters building, a company contracts for ongoing lawn care services. Several weeks later, the company nurse notes several severe skin rashes and an increasing frequency of gastrointestinal disorders among headquarters personnel. It is finally discovered that the lawn care contractor, while using a legally registered pesticide, applies the pesticide by broadcast spraying. This pesticide is known to cause severe allergenic reactions in sensitive humans, and also has toxic effects.

- *Item:* Did the plant audit include consideration of not only the health risks associated with operations conducted by plant personnel, but also by contractors?
- *Item:* Who, in addition to plant personnel, might have been exposed and what is company policy regarding the notification of such persons of their possible exposure?

Example 4.3   A company manufactures small metal parts by pressing metal dusts into molds under high pressure. The assembly line is composed mostly of young females. Neither plant uniforms nor hair nets are provided to machine operators. However, after an audit by the company's insurance company, the company decides to make it mandatory to wear paper dust masks for respiratory protection.

- *Item:* Did the audit consider the amount of toxic metal dust that might be carried home by plant personnel in their clothing and hair, or the possible subsequent exposure of the workers' children?

Example 4.4   Several chemical ingredients used in the manufacture of a plastic feed stock are extremely corrosive. The manufacturer has implemented an extensive and sophisticated set of control devices and procedures for controlling fumes from these chemical ingredients that might be released during accidental spills during delivery and the manufacturing process. A plant audit confirms that the various safety valves and backups, the computerized alarm system, and emergency response procedures are substantially more than adequate.

- *Item:* Did the audit consider the community risks due to tanker trucks carrying these corrosive chemicals to the plant along the public highway?
- *Item:* Are there constraints on the route taken by delivery tankers through the community based on particularly sensitive areas (e.g., hospitals, schools) or resources (e.g., drinking water supplies, groundwater recharge areas)?
- *Item:* What information has been provided to community authorities having responsibility for emergency response?

ELEMENTS OF THE HSE AUDIT

In integrating the real workplace into its real environment, it is necessary to examine the interactive physical, material, operational, procedural,

human, and informational aspects and attributes of both the workplace and
its environs.

Physical Aspects

Physical aspects to be considered include all constructed and naturally
occurring structural and physical features of the workplace and its environs
as well as their spatial relationships. Physical aspects include not only such
obvious structures as buildings, sheds, tanks, silos, transmission lines, containment dikes, reactor vessels, stacks, and roadways, but also such structures as underground pipes and conduits, landforms, groundwater aquifers,
unconsolidated soils, and surface water supplies.

While it is a relatively straightforward matter to define the physical
aspects of the workplace property, it is more difficult to define the geographic
extent to be considered beyond a company's property lines. The basic rule of
thumb is to encompass the *geographic area of actual risk*, which is essentially
any location that may (a) become a source of or contribute to an on-site
workplace hazard or (b) experience the risk of a hazard due to the workplace. For example, an off-site mosquito breeding ground can nonetheless
serve as a disease vector affecting the health of on-site workers, just as the
air emissions from one factory can be entrained in the ventilated air of a
distant factory. Similarly, on-site production of metallic dusts may result in
contamination of off-site water resources, with subsequent buildup of toxic
concentrations in aquatic food chains—a situation that can certainly affect
the health of even distant human populations that also participate in those
food chains.

There is no question that such a geographically comprehensive approach to defining the physical aspects of a company goes well beyond limits
of jurisdictional authority of an individual company, if not traditional limits
of legal responsibility. However, the fact remains that such a comprehensive
approach can be expected to soon become the norm in any serious HSE audit
of the workplace.

Material Aspects

"Material" means any physical, chemical, or biological substance or
agent that may pose a threat to human health and safety. These include
not only manufacturing feedstocks and wastes, but also products and by-
products of the manufacturing process. They also include environmentally
generated agents. For example, the ambient heat of the tropics poses as much
of a potentially threatening risk to a worker in the tropics as does excessive
heat produced by actual manufacturing processes in a temperate climate—

as, for example, in a foundry. In the process of working, it makes little difference to the health and safety of a worker should a particular risk be humanly or environmentally derived.

Often, a serious mistake is made by considering specific workplace materials as offering risk only to those workers whose job it is to handle those materials. Thus, for example, laboratory chemicals are usually considered in terms of the risks they present to laboratory technicians. However, laboratory chemicals can be carried home on contaminated clothing or entrained into make-up air that is ventilated to office workers.

Another common mistake is to assume that workplace materials obtained from retail sources (e.g., housekeeping supplies) can be safely ignored because, after all, they are products that people typically use at home. However, a retail product such as, say, a corrosive cleaner, may be used in the home only periodically and even then only for short periods of time, whereas, in the workplace, a person may use that same product continually throughout the workday.

A type of material of worldwide concern is, of course, blood and other bodily fluids that may be infected with the HIV or other viruses, such as the hepatitis virus. In workplaces that do not use blood or bodily fluids in production processes, the tendency is to ignore these materials. Yet, workplace accidents in any industry can, of course, expose company emergency response or health care personnel to these and other infectious agents.

Requiring a comprehensive inventory of the diverse materials brought into or generated within a plant, an HSE audit must clearly identify the diverse means whereby on-site personnel and the general public might become exposed to these materials. Essential to this task is a thorough examination of the various environmental dynamics (Chapter 2) associated with each material.

Operational Aspects

Plant operations include those activities undertaken as a direct consequence of production, including materials receiving, stockpiling and inventory control, in-plant distribution and transport of materials and products, production, quality control, maintenance, and shipping. Typically reflected in the departmental organizational structure of a company, plant operations are basically categorized by the essential, repetitive and highly coordinated activities that must be undertaken to turn raw stock materials into finished goods or, in the case of a service industry, to accomplish a contracted task.

Because operations are essentially coordinated actions directed toward specific goals, operations may easily be substructured into diverse *jobs*, *tasks*, and *skills*. A job is a category of responsibility for one or more operations, such as "laboratory technician." A person having a particular job usually has the responsibility for performing a number of different tasks. For example, a laboratory technician analyzes metal contamination of process water, makes up standard solutions, and maintains analytical notebooks and files. In undertaking individual tasks the laboratory technician has to exercise various skills, including weighing out chemicals, pipetting liquids, and calibrating instrumentation.

The analysis of a particular plant operation in terms of specific jobs and associated tasks and elements is often referred to in industry as *job analysis* or *operations analysis*. Only a comprehensive job analysis can provide the type of detailed information needed to identify the specific types of hazards the workplace presents to specific personnel. It is clearly not sufficient to know, for example, that someone "works in maintenance"; in order to identify the actual risks experienced by that worker, it is necessary to know specifically what, for working in the maintenance department, that particular worker has to do and the conditions under which the work has to be done.

Procedural Aspects

As step by step directions for accomplishing a specific task, procedural aspects of a comprehensive facility audit include not only those procedures for conducting production-oriented operations (e.g., how to charge a reactor vessel with a specific chemical reagent), but also those for accomplishing non-production-oriented tasks, such as notifying local emergency response organizations, reporting injuries to human resource personnel, and collecting and consolidating hazardous waste from satellite storage areas.

The importance of written procedures to an effective workplace health and safety program cannot be overemphasized. Not only do written procedures constrain workplace behavior to defined limits of risk, they also provide management with a rational basis for exerting quality control and oversight of the health and safety program, as well as provide regulatory authorities with evidence of good faith effort toward compliance.

With regard to potential litigation involving workplace injury, particularly serious attention should be given by upper level corporate management to that old adage: "if it doesn't exist on paper, it probably doesn't exist." Regrettably, companies that expend significant effort to document their activities in terms of written procedures beyond what may be required for regulatory compliance are in the vast minority. As corporations begin to understand that traditional limits of legal liability regarding both environmental quality and workplace health and safety are in fact becoming more and more irrelevant to jurisprudential, political, and social intent and expectations, it is likely that they will pay increasingly serious attention to developing written procedures for all activities that directly or indirectly impact HSE.

Human Aspects

The traditional facility audit typically restricted its attention to that specific category of humans known as "employee." Over the past decade, this term has become less inclusive of the persons who can be associated with a particular workplace, if only because of the well-established trend of companies differentiating between employees and so-called "temps"—members of the work force who are contracted from a service agency and who, as temporary workers at a plant, are not eligible for the benefits received by formal employees of that same plant.

While there are diverse economic and legal factors involved in this particular ongoing trend, it has tended to coincide with other trends, which may or may not be influenced by different factors, including the increasing use of on-site professional specialists who, as consultants, are actually employed by other corporations. To this contemporary workplace collage of employees, temps, and long-term on-site consultants must be added the traditional contractor who, either as a long-term or a short-term participant in the on-site activities of a modern corporation, is more and more frequently identified as of specific interest in regulations related to workplace health and safety.

The HSE audit expands this appreciation of persons who might experience health or safety risk due to the workplace still further to include:

- members of workers' households
- visitors to the workplace
- residential and other abutters to the facility's property
- persons providing public or private services, including local emergency response (e.g., fire and ambulance), mail, or other pick-up or delivery services
- any other member of the general public whose health or safety may be affected by the plant and associated activities (e.g., downstream receivers of air or water contaminants)

Just as it is necessary to determine how the worker may be exposed to an in-plant hazard, so it is necessary to determine (a) the precise mechanisms and means whereby the full range of persons whose health can be directly and indirectly associated with a company may experience risk due to that company, and (b) any characteristic or attribute of the potentially affected population (e.g., proximity of schoolchildren, downstream location of agricultural crops) that may exacerbate the risk.

Informational Aspects

A good rule of thumb for a site auditor is that the absence of on-site documented information directly or indirectly relevant to health and safety is probably a good measure of a company's dangerous disregard for human health and safety. However, of course, it is not just a question of what information is available, but also the ease with which it can be retrieved, the familiarity of workers and managers with the information, and evidence that the information has actually been used to achieve health and safety objectives.

Generic categories of information today considered essential to the design, implementation, and management of a comprehensive workplace health and safety program include, but are not necessarily limited to, the following:

- Up-to-date copies of regulations and pertinent health and safety standards
- Written documents required by specific regulations (e.g., accident reports, confined space entry programs, emergency response procedures, hazardous waste manifests, etc.)
- Documentation of health and safety risks associated with hazardous materials, including Material Safety Data Sheets (Chapter 5) and related scientific and technical publications
- Proceedings of meetings convened by the company safety committee or safety officer
- Description of all safety-related devices and equipment, including purpose, type, location, limits, and maintenance requirements
- Description of all personal protective clothing, including purpose type, task specificity, limits, and maintenance requirements
- Ambient monitoring records (for air and/or water)
- Safe operating specifications for equipment and devices
- Hazard and risk assessments of operations performed by facility personnel or by external consultants
- Inventory of hazardous materials, products, and by-products
- Evaluations and recommendations regarding health and safety incidents or conditions, as well as planned or implemented follow-up actions
- Personnel training records regarding any aspect of workplace health and safety, including names, dates, and subject matter

FINDINGS AND RECOMMENDATIONS

No audit that does not translate findings into specific recommendations for corporate action is worth the effort to perform. Regardless of the complexity of the facility audited and regardless of the many technical, scientific, and managerial issues that may be examined or become the object of concern, the HSE audit must finally and specifically address the following four primary questions:

1. What are the hazards that can be associated with this particular facility and all of its operations either on or off the property site?
2. What specific mechanisms or conditions either on- or off-site can mediate potential hazards into human health and safety risks?
3. Which on-site and off-site populations are at risk and what specific actions can be taken to mitigate the risks for each potentially affected population?
4. What type of quality control mechanism can be implemented to ensure the proper long-term management of selected mitigation measures?

PART II

HEALTH AND SAFETY PROGRAMS

CHAPTER 5

HAZARD COMMUNICATION

BACKGROUND

The Hazard Communication regulation, otherwise known in the United States as "Right-to-Know" (29 CFR 1910.1200) requires the development of a written program that addresses the worker's right to know:

1. What the Hazard Communication Standard is and what it requires,
2. What chemicals in the workplace are hazardous and what those hazards are,
3. How and where to obtain information about hazardous chemicals and how to use this information to ensure personal health and safety, and
4. What the employer is doing to ensure compliance with the Hazard Communication Standard.

In addressing these worker's rights, the written program (Table 5.1) must include procedures used by the company to determine chemical hazards, to employ labels and other forms of warning, to make available health and safety information regarding hazardous chemicals, and to conduct personnel training. Personnel training must include detailed information regarding the selection, proper use, and maintenance of personal protective clothing and equipment. Overall responsibility for the management of a hazard communication program that meets all requirements regarding the rights of personnel as well as personnel training must be assigned to a right-to-know coordinator (RTKC).

DETERMINATION OF HAZARDS

The regulation requires that the manufacturer of a chemical provide the user of that chemical with appropriate health and safety information.

TABLE 5.1   Major Topics to Be Included in a Written Hazard Communication Program

---

Hazard Communication Program
Table of Contents

1. Introduction
2. Overview of Program
3. Determination of Hazards
4. Labels and Other Forms of Warning
5. Material Safety Data Sheets (MSDSs)
6. Information and Training Program
7. Hazardous Chemicals
8. Hazards of Non-Routine Tasks
9. Chemicals in Unlabeled Pipes
10. Procedures for Contract Employees

Appendices

A. Inventory of Hazardous Chemicals
B. Employee Information & Training Program
    - OSHA Regulations
    - Operations Involving Hazardous Chemicals
    - Location & Availability of Hazard
        Communication Program
    - Detection of Hazardous Chemicals
    - Physical & Health Hazards
    - Protection from Hazardous Chemicals
    - Labels & Other Forms of Warning
    - Material Safety Data Sheets (MSDSs)

C. Technical Glossary

This information is to be provided in the form of a material safety data sheet (MSDS), which must be maintained by the company purchasing the relevant chemical and made available to company personnel.

While the intent of this requirement is to establish the MSDS provided by the chemical manufacturer as the basis for determining hazards and appropriate steps for ensuring the health and safety of those who might experience workplace exposure to the chemical, it is clear that the quality of MSDSs is highly variable. A key consideration is that a company's reliance on an MSDS is essentially reliance on the chemical manufacturer's word. While many chemical manufacturers expend significant effort to ensure the accuracy of their MSDSs, many do not—and a company's reliance upon information provided by the latter does not necessarily absolve a company from any legal liability regarding the use of inaccurate information.

A second major consideration regarding the determination of hazardous chemicals is the question of which chemicals fall within the purview of the standard. While there are various exemptions, such exemptions can be expected to vary among different nations. Some exemptions are open to diverse interpretation—as, for example, the exemption of a so-called "article" in the U.S. OSHA regulation. If sufficient guidance is not available in written regulations, it is always the wisest course to contact the responsible regulatory agency directly to clarify any confusion about legal exemptions.

Many corporate managers consider it most desirable to use a variety of strategies to make their inventory of in-plant chemical materials appear less hazardous than it actually is by relying on MSDSs that are either technically deficient or misleading, by selecting extremely narrow (if not convoluted or even preposterous) interpretations of legal exemptions, by equating the availability of a particular chemical substance through retail sources (e.g., paints, cleaners) with its "obvious" nonhazardous status, and even by using anecdotal, personal experience and so-called "common sense" to declare a particular chemical as nonhazardous. Such strategies are essentially counterproductive, both for managing workplace health and safety and for managing corporate legal liability. Typically, they are also in blatant contradiction with a basic tenet of toxicology, which is that any chemical may cause toxic effects if exposure to that chemical is sufficiently high.

Realistically, excellent measures of the basic good-faith corporate effort to protect personnel from chemical hazards are (a) the company's evident attempt to consider all potential chemical hazards and (b) the company's care in evaluating each chemical (or chemical mixture) with regard to potential hazards.

With regard to the in-plant use of MSDSs, the RTKC is well advised to establish an *MSDS Verification Procedure* as an attempt to verify the technical adequacy of any MSDS submitted to the company by a chemical manufacturer. One example of such a preliminary verification procedure is as follows:

1. If the MSDS identifies any pure chemical or mixture as hazardous, then that substance will be designated as hazardous.

2. If the MSDS identifies any pure chemical or mixture as nonhazardous, the RTKC will verify this evaluation before designating that pure chemical or mixture as nonhazardous.

3. The verification procedure shall consist of comparing the chemical name of the pure chemical or of each chemical in a mixture with chemical names included in standard references, which may include regulatory references (e.g., 29 CFR 1910 Subpart Z; the U.S. Registry of Toxic Effects of Chemical Substances), or commercially available references (e.g., handbooks of toxic and hazardous chemicals). Many references are available today in computerized as well as hard copy format, while e-mail capability through the World Wide Web (W^3) and modem access via remote login ensure essentially unlimited access to relevant information on chemical hazards.

4. If any chemical name that is included in these references as a hazardous chemical (and regardless of specified concentrations) is the same name (or its equivalent) of any chemical included in the chemical inventory, then that chemical will be designated as a hazardous chemical, even if the available MSDS declares it to be nonhazardous.

Given the broad availability of chemical information in CD-ROM format, it is advisable that the RTKC consider comparing the contents of MSDSs provided by company vendors with contents of MSDS available through commercial information vendors. Such a comparison is not appropriately included as a key step in an MSDS verification procedure.

The basic product of hazard determination is an inventory of chemicals (pure chemicals and mixtures) that clearly identifies for each chemical (a) the relevant hazard classes (Chapter 2), (b) potential routes of entry (i.e., ways in which a chemical can contact or enter the body), and (c) target organs (i.e., tissues or organs that are specifically affected by a hazardous chemical). Chemicals may typically be described in terms of multiple hazards, routes of entry, and target organs (Table 5.2), including any combination of the following:

A. **Hazard Classes** (definitions given in Chapter 2)
    • explosive • flammable • combustible • organic peroxide • pyrophoric • unstable/reactive • water reactive • oxidizer • asphyxiant • corrosive • irritant • sensitizer • poison • toxic • carcinogen • teratogen • mutagen • radioactive

B. **Routes of Entry**
    • inhalation • ingestion • surface contact • absorption • puncture

C. **Target Organs** (most commonly used; others are possible)
    • hair • skin • eye • ear • mucous membranes • lung • kidney • bladder • liver • gall bladder •

TABLE 5.2 Sample Page from a Chemical Inventory That Includes Chemically Specific Health and Safety Information

---

Global Enterprises, Inc.
Chemical Inventory

Department	Date	Authorization
Quality Control Laboratory	July 19, 1996	Elizabeth Kohl

1, 3-Phenylguanidine

Route(s): Inhalation; Absorption; Surface Contact
Hazard(s): Irritant; Sensitizer; Toxic
Target Organ(s): Skin; Eye; Mucous Membranes; Respiratory Tract

2-Butoxyethanol

Route(s): Inhalation; Ingestion; Absorption; Surface Contact
Hazard(s): Combustible; Irritant; Toxic; Teratogen
Target Organ(s): Skin; Eye; Mucous Membranes; Kidney; Liver; Blood; Respiratory Tract; Reproductive System; Lymphatic System

2, 4, 6-Trichlorophenol

Route(s): Inhalation; Ingestion; Absorption; Surface Contact
Hazard(s): Irritant; Toxic; Carcinogen
Target Organ(s): Skin; Eye; Mucous Membranes; Respiratory Tract

Acetophenetidin

Route(s): Inhalation; Ingestion; Absorption; Surface Contact
Hazard(s): Irritant; Toxic; Carcinogen; Teratogen; Mutagen
Target Organ(s): Skin; Eye; Mucous Membranes; Lung; Kidney; Bladder; Respiratory Tract, GI Tract; Reproductive System; Nervous System

Ceric Ammonium Nitrate

Route(s): Inhalation; Ingestion; Surface Contact
Hazard(s): Oxidizer; Irritant; Toxic
Target Organ(s): Skin; Eye; Mucous Membranes; Respiratory Tract

Page 3 of 65

pancreas • heart • spleen • blood • respiratory tract
• gastrointestinal tract • vascular system • reproductive
system • nervous system • lymphatic system • immunological system

Under no circumstances should the RTKC ignore any hazard, route
of entry, or target organ that is identified in a manufacturer's MSDS. However, the RTKC may add additional hazard classes, routes of entry, or target
organs that may be discovered on the basis of the verification procedure
discussed above.

Where a chemical substance is a mixture of chemicals and the mixture
has not been tested for health effects as a whole, the basic approach is to
describe the mixture in terms of the summation of hazards, routes of entry,
and target organs of each chemical constituent of the mixture.

LABELS AND OTHER FORMS OF WARNING

All containers of hazardous chemicals received from vendors should
be checked at the receiving dock to ensure that proper labels are attached.
Despite different requirements imposed by different legal jurisdictions, some
of which may pertain to print size, minimal information included on labels
typically includes:

1. Name of chemical (or product or trade name)
2. Appropriate hazard warning
3. Name and address of manufacturer (or importer)

Any vendor product that is not properly labeled should be returned
to the vendor unless urgent need for the product is determined. In such a
case, the RTKC should apply an in-plant label that includes the above information to the container. Labels, tags, or other markings affixed by the RTKC
should not deface or otherwise obscure labels or warnings affixed by the
manufacturer or importer.

It is important that the RTKC understand the differences in labels
that may be required for the transport of chemicals as opposed to those
required under health and safety regulations. In the United States, for example, labels or markings required for the transport of chemical containers
fall within the purview of the Hazardous Materials Transportation Act
(HMTA), which is administered by the U.S. Department of Transportation
(U.S. DOT), whereas labels or markings on in-plant containers are governed
by Occupational Safety and Health Act, which is administered by OSHA.

The requirements are quite different; compliance with one set of regulations does not imply compliance with the other.

To ensure the adequacy of labels, the RTKC is advised to computerize the chemical inventory, including the name of the chemical and appropriate hazards, routes of entry, and target organs as well as a code number that can be used to cross-reference inventory items with specific MSDSs. Sometimes a company will use a code number that also contains a purchasing or other inventory control number. Once computerized, this information can easily be used with any of numerous commercially available computer programs to generate in-plant labels.

In addition to providing for the adequacy of labels for chemical containers (including both primary and secondary containers), the RTKC is responsible for ensuring the signing of particular areas or structures, including (a) chemical storage areas, (b) pipes containing hazardous chemicals, (c) reactors, vessels, and other containers of chemicals presenting particularly acute hazards (e.g., flammability) or hazards requiring special precautions (e.g., water reactive or radioactive chemicals), and (d) areas presenting unusual hazards to external contractors (i.e., hazards not normally associated with a particular type of work environment).

The key issue with regard to any label, sign, or other visual warning is, of course, its intelligibility. This can be a particularly complex issue when the work force is composed of persons who speak different languages or are functionally illiterate. Different nations have, of course, different minimal requirements as to mandated languages used for labels and signs. In an effort to overcome the problems associated with a plural linguistic work force as well as functional illiteracy, many companies attempt to use so-called "universal symbols." Some companies use a combination of universal symbols, standardized color or numerical codes, and multiple-languaged warnings. Whatever the approach, the objective of "hazard communication" is to communicate—the RTKC must make a reasonable effort to ensure, either by appropriate physical means, personnel training, or both, that the worker in fact understands what warning labels, signs, and other types of communications (e.g., evacuation alarm signal) actually mean.

MANAGEMENT OF MATERIAL SAFETY DATA SHEETS

Beyond the verification of MSDSs (see Determination of Hazards, above) the workplace management of MSDSs requires careful consideration of several problematic issues, including (a) the timely procurement or, in some instances, the internal generation of an MSDS, (b) availability of the

MSDS to personnel, and (c) the integration of MSDSs with personnel training and other liaison activities.

Procurement

The basic rule is that no hazardous chemical should be in the workplace unless the RTKC has obtained an appropriate MSDS. This rule requires that purchasing agents coordinate with the RTKC to ensure that the company already has the appropriate MSDS or, in the case of a new chemical, that the company will receive the MSDS before the new chemical arrives at the loading dock. Otherwise, there is no way of implementing appropriate safety measures before the chemical arrives on-site.

To achieve this objective of the timely procurement of an MSDS, some companies require the RTKC to countersign each purchase of a chemical. In some companies, the generation of a purchase order is computer interlocked with the health and safety department. In the absence of such safeguards, other procedures have to be considered, including (a) confining all chemical deliveries until it can be verified as to whether or not the company does possess an appropriate MSDS and (b) requiring the in-house personnel who requested the item to demonstrate the in-house presence of an MSDS. Regardless of the real pressures of production schedules, which are frequently used to secure the release of an improperly documented hazardous chemical into the workplace, the widespread availability of fax machines and express mail delivery services precludes any excuse for not having required MSDSs readily provided by vendors.

Of course, chemicals enter into a workplace through means other than purchase orders. Chemicals are often mailed directly to personnel as samples. Sometimes, personnel bring chemicals from home into the plant. In many facilities, chemicals (especially cleaners, paints, and varnishes) can be bought at retail markets with petty cash or on the basis of personal cash reimbursement, thus precluding the generation of a purchase order. The RTKC must establish enforceable policies to ensure that chemicals entering the workplace through such means are properly documented by an MSDS.

Some chemicals enter the workplace because they are generated as by-products of plant operations. In such a case, it becomes the responsibility of the RTKC to generate the appropriate MSDS, using either in-house personnel or external consultants.

Some chemicals enter the workplace simply because they are brought onto company property by contractors. The company must therefore ensure that no contractor bring any hazardous chemical on-site except by express permission of the RTKC. Permission should be denied if appropriate MSDSs are not immediately available. This is often accomplished today by requiring contractors to identify any of their hazardous chemicals during a sign-in procedure, prior to their entry to the workplace.

Finally, hazardous chemicals can be transmitted to the workplace from remote locations through ambient air, water, or dust. While this is a particularly problematic issue because of the multiple sources possibly involved (e.g., exhausts of highway vehicles) and the lack of identifiable authority or jurisdiction, the RTKC does have certain recourses, including:

1. Minimizing entry to the workplace through the use of protective equipment and devices (e.g., installing absorbent filters in air intakes) and
2. Implementing an ambient monitoring program that is integrated with automatic alarm systems, including evacuation alarms.

Even where such measures substantially reduce the risk of externally derived hazards, and even should the risk be well within promulgated standards, the RTKC should consider developing generic MSDSs, which summarize the health and safety information relevant to common, so-called "environmental hazards," such as vehicular exhausts, dusts, organic vapors, and agricultural pesticides.

Availability to Personnel

While MSDSs are intended to be available to facility personnel at all times, some practical problems typically result in bureaucratic obstacles to access. For example, some companies require personnel to complete a standard "request form" that is subsequently acted upon by the plant safety officer. This is usually an attempt to document or otherwise manage the flow of paper in the plant by preventing spurious requests. Some companies insist that personnel personally request an MSDS from the human resource manager or a regulatory compliance officer—again, purportedly to introduce some measure of management over what is often perceived of as a process that, if not controlled, may result in inordinate time spent on searching files, photocopying, or controlling potential sensitive company information.

Despite such arguments, which themselves seem most often spurious or at least reflective of a corporate preoccupation with bureaucratic process, and even sometimes clearly indicative of a corporate attempt to identify potential trouble makers, the MSDS is intended primarily as a source of information, not only to managers but to personnel who work with chemicals. Any policy or procedure that in any way impedes immediate access to this information by employees should be suspected as contrary to the intent of right-to-know regulations and carefully reconsidered.

The ideal situation is one in which MSDSs are freely and immediately available in the various work areas of a plant or, if located in a centralized area, located so that workers have direct access without having to ask permission or otherwise delay their access by having to change out of work clothes, incur the trouble of travel from one building to another, or set up an appointment.

It is understood, of course, that timely access to MSDSs is itself not enough. Personnel must have equal access to any reference materials, such as technical glossaries or other descriptive materials, that can facilitate their understanding of information contained in MSDSs.

In instances in which a worker may desire a personal take-home copy of an MSDS, it is certainly understandable that a company may opt to exercise control over the economics of photocopying MSDSs. After all, a typical manufacturing company may have a chemical inventory of one to several thousand MSDSs and simply cannot undertake to provide every employee with personal copies of MSDSs, each of which may contain several to a dozen or more pages.

Integration with Training and Other Activities

In the United States and in other nations where workplace safety may be regulated at state as well as Federal levels, different regulatory agencies promulgate different requirements regarding the specific manner in which MSDSs are integrated with personnel training, liaison with governmental agencies, and coordination with local emergency response services.

Over and above specific requirements, it is generally to be recommended that MSDSs be assigned distinct identification codes that can easily be incorporated in all subsequent in-house training on hazardous chemicals. The reason for this is that MSDSs typically vary greatly with regard to the format in which information is presented. Immediate comprehension of even the identity of the chemical is often impossible due to the diverse practices regarding the use of chemical, product, or brand-names, as well as the use of numerous chemical synonyms. The most prominent name for acetone in a particular MSDS, for example, may be "acetone," or "dimethyl ketone," or "2-propanone," or even something like "wonder solvent super-X" or "S66." Distinct codes, including so-called "part numbers" and purchasing codes avoid confusion due to the frequent plurality of names of workplace chemicals and greatly facilitate immediate access to relevant information. All in-plant communications regarding a specific chemical, especially training materials, labels, and warning signs, computerized or hard copies of chemical inventories, and requirements for personal protective clothing and equipment should include prominent reference to the relevant unique code for that chemical.

Regarding liaison with external authorities and services (e.g., emergency response services), additional coding may be considered. For example, it is common for fire chiefs in the United States to require that chemicals be assigned the number and color designations assigned to chemicals by the National Fire Prevention Association (NFPA) or those codes used in commonly consulted manuals, such as the U.S. Department of Transportation's Emergency Response Manual. A variety of other coding systems, known as *hazardous materials information systems* (HMIS), are generally available, including systems employing colors, numbers, alpha-numerics, and key words.

PERSONNEL TRAINING

Categorical requirements for personnel training include the following:

1. The requirements of pertinent Right-to-Know regulation,
2. The identification of operations conducted in any work area where hazardous chemicals are present,
3. The location and availability of the written Hazard Communication Program, including the list of hazardous chemicals and MSDSs,
4. Methods and observations that may be used to detect the presence or release of a hazardous chemical,
5. The physical and health hazards of chemicals,
6. The measures that employees can take to protect themselves from chemical hazards, including specific procedures for protecting against exposure, appropriate work practices, emergency procedures, and the use of personal protective clothing and equipment, and
7. The details of the written Hazard Communication Program, including an explanation of the labeling system and MSDSs and how employees can obtain and use the appropriate information on hazards, health, and safety.

All employees and temporary contracted personnel (temps) who may reasonably be expected to come into contact with hazardous chemicals, either through normal work activities or through foreseeable emergencies (fire, explosion, flood, etc.), must receive training prior to their job assignment. Subsequent training must be given whenever a new hazard is introduced into the workplace or upon reassignment of personnel to new work areas.

In determining training needs, it is particularly important that the hazards of nonroutine tasks be considered in addition to normal and emergency operations. Nonroutine tasks include those tasks that do not relate directly to the manufacture of products or to normal daily or emergency operations of the plant, including periodic plant shut-downs, major refurbishing or construction, and significant alteration of plant procedures.

Contractors

Given the health and safety hazards possibly experienced by or derived through the activities of on-site contractors, the growing regulatory attention given to contractors, and the potential legal liabilities involved, companies are today beginning to give special attention to the training given to contractors regarding hazard communication.

While most contractors are typically quick to give assurance that they have received appropriate hazard communication training from their own corporation, the purchaser of contractor services is well advised to consult legal counsel to determine appropriate instruments for assuring verification of training. In some instances, companies require the contractor to agree to training stipulations within the contract prior to undertaking any on-site work; some companies require the contractor to provide other written documentation.

Increasingly, companies require the RTKC to follow a formal process for determining any special training needs of potential contractors. This process generally commits the RTKC to:

1. Identify all chemical health and safety hazards to which the contractor may reasonably be expected to be exposed in the performance of the contracted work,
2. Provide the contractor with a clear, documented explanation of the hazards and ensure the contractor's access to appropriate MSDSs,
3. Provide the contractor with a clear, documented explanation of relevant company safety and emergency response procedures,
4. Evaluate the appropriateness of the contractor's protective clothing and equipment and, as necessary, provide or require the contractor to obtain appropriate protective clothing and equipment, and
5. Obtain the contractor's written verification that the contractor received all necessary information and guidance to undertake the work without unwarranted exposure to workplace chemical hazards.

Records

While the design and implementation of the employee information and training program is generally the overall responsibility of the RTKC, other personnel, including human resource personnel, in-plant trainers, and external training consultants, may play key roles. Specific responsibility should be assigned for maintaining a log (written or computerized) of all training activities as well as a file of training materials and of the qualifications of external training consultants. Many companies require employees to sign off for each training session that they attend.

It is today very common that training records include the results of written or oral tests taken by personnel in the progress of their training. Where testing or examination of employees is employed, it is necessary not only to maintain copies of completed tests, but also written records of the tests themselves, the criteria for measuring performance, and any follow-up actions taken regarding an employee's failure to meet the test criteria.

Information regarding the hazard assessment made of normal, emergency, and nonroutine operations also must be maintained, including:

- description of normal, emergency, and nonroutine operations
- description of chemical hazards associated with each operation
- identification of personnel directly or possibly involved or exposed
- safety procedures to be implemented with respect to each operation
- safety equipment and supplies required for each operation
- description of instructions and training to be given to personnel prior to conducting each operation
- procedures for reviewing a potential health or safety incident

Finally, a record must also be maintained of any contractor's verification regarding hazard communication training received on- or off-site, as well as verification that the contractor has not brought any hazardous chemical into the facility except with the express permission of the RTKC (or the RTKC's delegate authority), which permission cannot be granted without the immediate availability of the relevant MSDSs.

While various regulations may specify time requirements for maintaining particular training records, the best advice is to maintain all training related files for the duration of the company's existence.

Performance Standard

A *performance standard* measures success in terms of actual job performance or, in other words, the actual behavior of personnel, as opposed to a *compliance standard*, which measures success in terms of following written directions. It is, therefore, quite possible to have a training program that meets the letter of the law, but which is also totally ineffectual in altering on-the-job performance.

Training undertaken to meet the objectives of hazard communication must be performance oriented. It is not sufficient that the company simply show films, distribute training materials, or put up warning signs. Communication is not synonymous with lecturing nor, as evidenced by the significant number of functional illiterates in possession of a college degree, is learning equivalent to having been inundated with information.

The measure of successful training in hazard communication is the degree to which personnel actually translate health and safety information into daily workplace behavior—which is, it must be reiterated, not an easily accomplished objective nor one, certainly, to be casually entrusted to the whims of essentially unqualified or disinterested training personnel. Basic guidelines for ensuring a successful, performance-oriented training program regarding hazard communication include:

1. Training must be based on a detailed job analysis that includes not only job tasks related to normal production operations, but also to emergencies, nonroutine operations, and the activities of contractors. Descriptions of job tasks must give particular emphasis to (a) actions that have to be undertaken by employees and (b) the specific information required by the employee to perform those actions.

2. Training objectives must be stated in terms of precisely how the employee is to demonstrate what is to be learned as a result of the training—i.e., training objectives must be action-oriented. It is not sufficient, for example, to state that the employee will understand the importance of wearing protective gloves. The action-oriented training objective is, rather, that the employee will be able to demonstrate how to use a glove-selection chart to select the proper type of glove to wear when handling a variety of in-plant corrosives and skin-absorbable chemicals.

3. The learning situation must simulate actual job tasks as closely as possible, with particular attention given to the sequence of actions that must be followed in performing individual tasks. While having some utility with regard to certain training objectives, the generic packaging of information through commercially available films and booklets and "off-the-shelf" lectures by consultants typically cannot by themselves provide the necessary job and plant specificity required for effective, performance-oriented training. Such training materials and mechanisms must be carefully supplemented and orchestrated by in-plant experience.

4. Performance-oriented training can be effectively evaluated only through the follow-up assessment of actual job performance. Regardless of the evident high level of sophistication of training materials or presenters, no

training can be considered worth the effort if it does not actually result in enhanced on-the-job safety. Failures in achieving behavioral objectives are failures in training and in the managerial enforcement of training objectives.

Given the time and effort that must be expended in designing and implementing effective performance-oriented training, the importance of the support and interest of upper-level corporate management cannot be overemphasized. The level of corporate support and interest must, after all, reflect not only the human concern of plant owners and executives for the health and safety of their employees, but also their recognition of corporate and personal legal liabilities that are increasingly engendered by all too frequent training failures.

Selected Substantive Issues

Among the various substantive issues that must be addressed by the Hazard Communication Standard, several are particularly problematic and deserve particular attention, including (a) the detection of hazardous chemicals, (b) acute and chronic health effects, and (c) protective clothing, equipment, and procedures.

Detection of Hazardous Chemicals

Because personnel training under the Hazard Communication Standard must include specific information on the means whereby hazardous chemicals may be detected, personnel training typically includes consideration of ambient air monitoring and, less frequently, of signs and symptoms of chemical exposure.

Ambient monitoring is discussed in detail in Chapter 16. It is therefore sufficient here to emphasize that, with regard to the training aspect of ambient monitoring, the RTKC is probably best advised to use the manufacturer of each chosen monitoring device to train in-plant personnel in the proper use and maintenance of that device. This approach will not only ensure that training will be conducted by persons having the greatest familiarity with monitoring devices, but also likely provide the greatest corporate protection regarding potential legal liability associated with the technical conduct of ambient monitoring. All in-plant personnel should, of course, receive training in all aspects of an ambient monitoring program, including regulatory requirements, the selection of parameters and devices, the meaning and significance of monitoring data, and actions to be implemented should monitored levels exceed recommended limits or standards.

The issue of human symptomatology with regard to chemical exposure is generally considered a sensitive issue by companies because of the simple fact that the symptoms of chemical exposure in the workplace include precisely all the symptoms of human health that are generally associated with non-work-related exposures, disease, and even personal behavior. Headaches, after all, may reflect exposure to an industrial organic solvent, a flu, or a hangover.

Despite the nonspecificity of human health symptoms, their potential value as a workplace alert to hazardous conditions should be carefully considered, particularly in those instances in which a number of personnel in the same work environment exhibit similar symptoms.

Just as most companies have become quite used to the formal reporting of even minor physical injuries such as cuts, abrasions, and muscle strain to their insurance underwriters, more and more companies are beginning to implement a formal reporting of symptoms such as dizziness, coughing, stinging or redness of eyes, diarrhea, and tightness in chest as potential signs of exposure to workplace chemicals—this despite the fact that many executives persist in arguing that this approach is tantamount to blaming the workplace for the consequences of common ailments that have nothing to do with the workplace.

A proper emphasis on human symptomatology, which underscores its real limits as a means of identifying the definite cause of apparently minor health ailments, is nonetheless of inestimable value as an alert to potential workplace hazards that, if ignored, might result in significant injury. One objective of training under hazard communication should therefore be the ability of employees to identify typical health symptoms that can be associated with exposures to specific workplace chemicals, among other possible causes.

Hazard Classes

Even though the general public has become increasingly aware of the fact that many health effects of chemical exposures can take years and even decades to become evident, the concern for chemical safety in the workplace still tends to be dominated by a consideration of the acute effects of relatively large exposures to chemicals as opposed to chronic effects, especially of low exposures. This tendency is often exacerbated by social and cultural factors, including the competition for employment, which gives priority to personal income over personal health; male machismo, which denies any outward sign of fear or concern; the natural ebullience of youth, which fosters a sense of indestructibility; and even sometimes by a cultural stoicism, which elevates impassiveness to pain and suffering to a virtue. In fact, this tendency is all too often promoted by a corporate management that profits economically from the willingness of employees to endure needless risk. This tendency, of course, also derives in large part from simple ignorance about the long-term effects of chemical exposure.

Any training program that seriously attempts to impact positively workplace health and safety must be based upon the balanced recognition of acute and chronic health effects of chemicals as well as upon the recognition that, while some health effects may be experienced by current employees, other effects, including mutational and developmental effects, may be passed on to their children.

Protective Clothing, Equipment, and Procedures

While training under the Hazard Communication Standard must address the personal protective clothing and equipment, important failings are common, including:

- failure to emphasize that each item of protective clothing (e.g., protective gloves) and of personal protective equipment (e.g., a respirator) has specific limitations—that none gives universal protection
- failure to emphasize the proper care and maintenance of protective clothing and equipment, including distinctive signs of wear, dysfunction, or impairment
- failure to identify personal factors that can negate the proper use of specific protective items, such as facial hair or the physical contour of the face that might preclude a worker's wearing a respirator
- failure to specify spatial restrictions regarding the wearing of certain items, such as a smock, which may protect a worker from dusts in the work area but which can contaminate food when worn in the cafeteria

Major failings are also common regarding personnel training in those procedures specifically designed to minimize chemical exposures, including procedures related to:

- the disposal of chemicals into sinks, especially where sink drains empty to on-site disposal systems that can contaminate local ground water supplies
- the storage of incompatible or reactive chemicals that can result in the generation of fire, explosion, and toxic fumes
- the transport of hazardous chemicals along routes through the plant where there is insufficient means for emergency containment

or where employees work who do not have required personal protective equipment (e.g., office staff)
- the restriction of plant visitors to protected areas
- the distribution of mail containing chemical samples
- personal dress codes (or the lack thereof) that can result, for example, in the exposure of bare legs and feet to hazardous chemicals

CHAPTER 6

LABORATORY STANDARD

BACKGROUND

Essentially a "Right-to-Know" standard specifically adapted for use in laboratories, the Laboratory Standard includes many requirements identical to the Hazard Communication Standard, including requirements related to the determination of chemical hazards, the use of MSDSs, the training of personnel, and the rights of employees to information regarding workplace hazards and means for protecting themselves from exposure. The reader should therefore consult Chapter 5 when reading this chapter.

In the United States, the exemption of laboratories from the Hazard Communication Standards was at first commonly attributed to Federal recognition that laboratory personnel are much more knowledgeable about chemical safety than employees in other industries. This understanding is blatantly wrong. By promulgating the Laboratory Standard (29 CFR 1910.1450), OSHA reiterated a special concern for health and safety in the laboratory, a concern predicated on the fact that laboratory exposures to chemicals are basically different from exposures in other industries because the former typically involve a larger number of different chemicals and also smaller doses.

Precisely because we are profoundly ignorant of the potential chronic health effects of low-level, essentially simultaneous exposures to the many different chemicals generally found in laboratories, the Laboratory Standard differs from the Hazard Communication Standard in its more expanded and explicit emphasis on written procedures for controlling chemical exposure and the medical surveillance of laboratory personnel (Table 6.1). As experience with the Laboratory Standard increases, it is highly probable that a comparable emphasis on written procedures and medical surveillance will be incorporated into the Hazard Communication Standard.

Overall responsibility for compliance with the Laboratory Standard is assigned to an in-house chemical hygiene officer (CHO). In small compa-

Chemical Hygiene Plan
Table of Contents

1. **Introduction**

2. **Responsibility**

3. **Standard Operating Procedures: General**

   - Personal Preparation & Behavior
   - Preparation of Work Area & Equipment
   - Maintenance of Work Area
   - Emergencies
   - Ordering Chemicals
   - Receiving Chemicals
   - Transporting Chemicals
   - Storing Chemicals
   - Using Laboratory Chemicals
   - Using Extremely Hazardous Chemicals

4. **Standard Operating Procedures: Chemically Specific**

   - Compressed Gases
   - Corrosive Chemicals
   - Flammable Chemicals
   - Extremely Hazardous Chemicals
   - OSHA Listed Chemicals

5. **Methods for Limiting Exposure**

   - Engineering Controls
   - Fume Hood Inspection
   - Personal Protective Clothing & Equipment
   - Emergency Equipment

6. **Availability of Data & Information**

7. **Personnel Training**

8. **Medical Surveillance**

   - Exposure Determination
   - Methods of Surveillance
   - Documentation

9. **Determination of Health Hazards**

   - Acute Hazards
   - Chronic Hazards

10. **Special Issues**

    - Prior Approval for New Chemicals
    - Chemicals Generated in Laboratory

Appendices

nies that must comply with both the Laboratory Standard and the Hazard Communication Standard, a safety officer often fills the roles of both the CHO and right-to-know coordinator (RTKC); in large companies, these roles are frequently undertaken by different employees. While, historically, the CHO has been selected from among laboratory personnel, many companies have found it more desirable to utilize nonlaboratory personnel (e.g., a corporate regulatory compliance officer, a plant operations manager) in the position of CHO. This approach has usually been taken in order to avoid what is perceived as a strong reluctance among scientifically trained personnel to alter historically defined ways of doing laboratory work.

In conformance with a recommendation included in the Laboratory Standard, many companies have opted to establish a chemical hygiene committee (CHC) or a safety committee to provide technical and administrative support to the CHO. In such instances it is advisable that such a committee include legal counsel and corporate officers as well as technical personnel. Laboratory managers, the hazardous waste coordinator (HWC), and the plant maintenance supervisor should also be included.

STANDARD OPERATING PROCEDURES

Written standard operating procedures (SOPs) have long been procedural fixtures in the typical laboratory as the basic means of ensuring scientific (if not regulatory) compliance with standardized analytical techniques, procedures, and protocols. The Laboratory Standard expands this meaning of SOPs to include health and safety procedures, historically known as *prudent practices*, that have previously been simply advisory or nonbinding. Under this standard, health- and safety-oriented SOPs are of two types: (a) general SOPs, which focus on generic issues that pertain to all laboratories, and (b) specific SOPs, which focus on the particular kinds of chemical hazards present in a particular laboratory.

General SOPs

General SOPs are written procedures and policies designed to minimize the health and safety risks by focusing on such universal aspects of laboratory work as:

- personal preparation and behavior of laboratory personnel
- preparation of the work area and equipment
- maintenance of the work area
- emergencies

- ordering chemicals
- receiving chemicals
- transporting chemicals
- storing chemicals
- using chemicals
- disposing of chemicals
- labeling chemical containers

Site Specificity

While the technical and scientific literature offers many examples of prudent practices regarding these issues, what is in fact prudent in a particular laboratory depends upon the specifics of that laboratory in terms of the types of analyses performed, chemical inventory, layout, and the potential health and safety hazards. Therefore, even general SOPs must be based on a comprehensive site evaluation (or hazard assessment) of the actual laboratory.

For example, while "familiarizing oneself with a reagent before using it" is a universally recognized prudent practice, including such a requirement in a general SOP regarding personal preparation may be quite insufficient in a particular laboratory in which highly reactive or unstable reagents are used. In such a case, the more prudent SOP may require written verification that the technician has consulted specific technical information about a reagent (e.g., boiling point, vapor pressure, upper and lower explosion level) before the technician is even granted access to that chemical.

Another example of a common failure to consider the potential ramifications of general SOPs in terms of site-specific details is the frequent misuse of lab coats. While it is certainly prudent laboratory practice to wear a lab coat, an SOP that simply requires the wearing of a lab coat is not only frequently of negligible value, but can even be counterproductive to health and safety. For example, lab coats worn over shorts are of highly questionable value in a laboratory in which highly corrosive materials are commonly used. A lab coat worn in a pathology laboratory by a technician who performs gross preparation of potentially infectious tissue and then worn to the bathroom or cafeteria can easily become a disease vector among not only other laboratory personnel but also the general public.

Extremely Hazardous Chemicals

In addition to site-specific factors, general SOPs must also be informed by specific requirements of the Laboratory Standard, including requirements for the identification, labeling, and storage of *extremely hazardous chemicals*. There is widespread confusion as to the phrase extremely hazardous chemical because the experiential understanding of "extremely hazardous" does not correspond to the regulatory definition.

Under the American OSHA Laboratory Standard, an extremely hazardous chemical has any one or more of the following three characteristics:

1. It has high acute toxicity (i.e., based on its LD_{50} [Chapter 3], it is a "poison")
2. It is a reproductive toxin, which means it has mutagenic or teratogenic effects or otherwise affects the human reproductive system
3. It is a "select carcinogen," meaning

    A. It is regulated by U.S. OSHA as a carcinogen, or
    B. It is listed under the category "known to be carcinogens" in the Annual Report on Carcinogens published by the U.S. National Toxicology Program (NTP), or
    C. It is listed under Group 1 ("carcinogenic to humans") by the International Agency for Research on Cancer (IARC) Monographs, or
    D. It is listed under IARC as Group 2A (at least limited evidence of carcinogenicity in humans) or Group 2B (sufficient evidence of carcinogenicity in animals) or is described by NTP as "reasonably anticipated to be carcinogenic" and causes statistically significant tumor incidence in experimental animals in accordance with U.S. OSHA specified criteria.

By this definition, sulfuric acid is not an extremely hazardous chemical under the Laboratory Standard, even though it is, in fact, extremely hazardous. The key difference between regulatory and nonregulatory meanings is that the focus of the OSHA regulation is on particular types of toxicity, including acute lethality, and selected chronic toxicities (reproductive and carcinogenic) that may result even from very small doses.

Under the Laboratory Standard, extremely hazardous chemicals must be identified and labeled as such. A general SOP, one that easily qualifies as a recognized prudent practice, might be stated as: "Do not modify the manufacturer's label on any chemical container." However, in light of the Laboratory Standard, the more prudent SOP might be phrased accordingly: "If the chemical requires additional labeling as an extremely hazardous chemical, attach the label to the container without obscuring any portion of the label provided by the manufacturer."

These examples clearly demonstrate that even general laboratory SOPs must be devised and implemented only on the basis of a comprehensive understanding of the actual hazards and risks presented by the individual laboratory—which can be determined only by means of a thorough audit (Chapter 4)—and of the precise requirements of the Laboratory Standard.

Specific SOPs

Other SOPs include those that are specific to (a) individual types of chemicals, such as flammables, corrosives, and extremely hazardous chemicals, and (b) particular requirements for limiting human exposure to laboratory hazards, such as personal protective clothing and equipment, fume hoods, and emergency equipment.

Chemicals

Whereas a general SOP regarding the handling, storage, or transport of chemicals will typically focus on generic concerns, such as leaking containers, chemical compatibility of stored chemicals, and the use of secondary containers, more detailed SOPs are required for the safe handling, storage, or transport of particular kinds of chemicals.

For example, to minimize the potential for accidental explosion, some chemicals that form peroxides upon standing should be discarded after 12 months (e.g., acrylic acid, cyclohexene, methylacetylene); others, after 3 months (e.g., isopropyl ether, vinylidene chloride, divinyl acetylene). While it is always good practice with regard to long-term chemical storage to separate oxidizers (which promote burning) and combustible chemicals (which can be ignited) it is often necessary to specify restrictions on even temporary, on-the-bench storage—as in disallowing the presence of certain oxidizers (e.g., chromic acid, hydrobromic acid, nitric acid) and certain highly flammable organic chemicals (e.g., acetone, petroleum ether) on the same bench, except for specified operational purposes or in limited amounts.

In some cases, such as where accidentally spilled or mixed chemicals may combine to produce an immediate threat to life or health (e.g., the production of cyanide gas or hydrogen sulfide), prudent practice may require absolute restrictions on the spatial separation of reactive chemicals (e.g., fuming nitric acid and acetic acid), regardless of volume.

Protective Clothing and Equipment

The formulation of SOPs regarding personal protective clothing and equipment also requires careful attention to detail. For example, the distinction between the need for safety glasses or for goggles must be premised upon the distinction between protection from impact to the eye, which is afforded by safety glasses, and infusion to the eye of dusts, mists and vapors, which is afforded by goggles. However, goggles are variously vented, with superior, inferior, medial or even radial locations (with respect to the lens) offering more or less protection depending upon whether dusts, mists, or vapors are likely in a particular situation to rise or fall toward the eye.

Even after 6 years' experience with the Laboratory Standard, typical SOPs regarding the use of protective gloves are often sorely deficient. In all too many laboratories, only gloves used for home dishwashing are available—oftentimes because company purchasing agents are ever on the lookout for bargains.

A proper SOP regarding the use of protective gloves must be based on the completion of the following key tasks:

1. The chemical inventory is reviewed to identify those chemicals that are corrosives, irritants, sensitizers, or skin-absorbable.

2. Each laboratory operation involving each of these chemicals is examined with regard to limits imposed by the need for manual dexterity.

3. Based on the names of chemicals and limits on dexterity, the information provided by glove manufacturer is consulted to identify (a) appropriate types of gloves, (b) the limits of protection afforded by each type in terms of the degree of protection and time duration, and (c) the proper use, maintenance, and replacement requirements associated with each type.

4. Once appropriate gloves are selected, relevant SOPs are established to ensure each laboratory operation identified on the basis of hazard (item 1, above) is conducted by personnel who understand and follow the written directions for obtaining, using, maintaining, and replacing the appropriate type of glove.

Fume Hoods

The Laboratory Standard gives particular emphasis to fume hoods, which are, after all, the most common means of managing human exposure to hazardous materials in laboratories. Because fume hoods are so common in laboratories, their efficacy with regard to health and safety is, unfortunately, often taken for granted—as is manifest by the rather abbreviated attention they are given in SOPs governing their use and maintenance in the industrial laboratory. Typical failures in SOPs include:

- the failure to specify that the fume hood is not to be used for the storage of chemicals but, rather, for operations that cannot be performed in the ambient atmosphere without undue risk
- the failure to prevent the use of unprotected live electrical terminals or circuits (e.g., plugs, heating coils, open coil motors, etc.) within fume hoods used for operations involving explosive, flammable, or combustible reagents
- the failure to assess potential risks engendered by the structural design of the hood, which may allow flammable or corrosive fumes to migrate from below-hood storage shelves (often wrongly used

for chemical storage) into behind-hood raceways containing electrical conduits

- the failure to determine and manage hood face velocity with regard to variable sash height, air make-up requirements of laboratory ventilation, and specific chemical operations conducted in the hood
- the failure to implement a regularly scheduled and rigorous fume hood inspection, which includes at least an annual inspection of all associated ducts, motors and belts, as well as the potential for hood exhaust to become entrained in ventilation intakes
- the failure to implement a regularly scheduled (usually annual) cleaning of hood ducts and exhaust conduits that can concentrate hazardous and even reactive chemicals
- the failure to establish requirements for personal protective clothing and equipment to be used during the inspection and cleaning of hoods
- the failure, regarding the use of mobile hoods, to establish clear protocols for the scheduled replacement of filter materials or to establish the requirement for "bag-in, bag-out" capability

Format and Location of SOPs

Depending upon the industry, different laboratories have different requirements regarding the format of written SOPs; sometimes these formats are based on regulatory requirements (e.g., food and drug regulations), and sometimes on long established corporate policy. Generally, the most useful SOPs are concise—they fit easily on a page and thereby provide easy and rapid access to precise information.

The particular format aside, it is abundantly clear that the compilation of SOPs into large notebooks results in cumbersome tomes that are counterproductive to frequent consultation. Ideally, the SOP should be as close to the operation it governs as possible. For example, the written scientific SOPs that an analytical laboratory uses on a daily basis to prepare solutions or conduct measurements and other analytical operations are ideal locations for relevant health and safety information. This approach ensures that when a laboratory technician follows a written analytical SOP, that technician also follows the directions of a written health and safety SOP directly relevant to the operation being performed. Of course, cross-referenced, computerized SOPs are probably the best means of assuring immediate access to the health and safety aspects of laboratory operations and procedures. When specific apparatus or equipment (e.g., a fume hood) is dedicated to a particular operation, it is advisable that the appropriate health and safety SOP be located in the immediate vicinity.

MEDICAL SURVEILLANCE

Under the American Laboratory Standard, laboratory workers have a right to medical consultations and examinations whenever:

1. The employee is known to have experienced exposure above (a) the *action level* of a particular chemical, which is a concentration designated in 29 CFR 1910 for a specific substance or, in the absence of an action level, (b) the OSHA promulgated threshold limit value (TLV; Chapter 3), or

2. There is a spill, leak, explosion or other emergency resulting in potential exposure of employees to any hazardous chemical, or

3. An employee may develop signs or symptoms that might be associated with an exposure to laboratory chemicals.

The first trigger presumes that the CHO has (a) determined specifically which chemicals in the laboratory inventory are regulated with respect to action level and/or a TLV and (b) implemented an appropriate ambient monitoring program for regulated chemicals. The second trigger presumes that the CHO has implemented a comprehensive emergency response program. The third trigger presumes that the CHO has established precise correlations between laboratory chemicals and potential human symptomatology. Of course, the overriding assumption of all three is that personnel have been adequately informed of their right to medical consultation and examination.

All medical consultations and examinations must be performed by or under the direct supervision of a licensed physician and must be provided by the company to the employee without cost to the employee and without loss of pay.

In order to ensure a proper medical surveillance program the CHO will not only have to have completed the tasks implicit in the above triggers, but also additional tasks that directly affect the adequacy of the program, including:

Selection of Medical Facility

To date, and certainly depending upon location, there are relatively few medical facilities having specific experience with industrial exposures. Where possible, the CHO should give primary consideration to those facilities and medical personnel that have industrial experience and have diagnostic and clinical capabilities that are commensurate with the specific types of chemicals present in the laboratory. Some companies have found it necessary to supplement the wherewithal of a responding medical facility by donating specific equipment and supplies (e.g., antidotes) to that facility. Other key considerations include the timeliness of access to the medical facility, including the availability of ambulances and medivac helicopters, the total number of potentially exposed personnel that may have to be examined at the same time, and, in less time-constrained circumstances, the general ease of access by individual employees. Upon selection of an appropriate facility, many companies attempt to establish a contractual relationship with the medical facility.

Providing Information

As soon as a medical facility is selected, the CHO is best advised to ensure that the facility is provided with a continually updated copy of the laboratory's chemical inventory, which should include not only the chemical name (of the pure chemical or, for a mixture, of each chemical ingredient) but also, for each item, (a) potential hazards, (b) routes of entry, and (c) target organs. Ideally, the CHO will have reviewed this information with a potential facility during the facility selection process in order to evaluate the relevant capability of the facility.

Additional information should be provided at the time of each incident requiring medical surveillance. This information, which is often provided in the format of a corporate form, includes:

- Name of employee
- Date of exposure incident (actual or potential)
- Names of chemicals involved in incident
- MSDSs (attached) for each chemical substance possibly involved
- Potential exposure data (values/units/dates)
- Mode of personnel exposure (e.g., inhalation) or related circumstances (e.g., fire)
- Signs or symptoms of exposure as shown by employee (description, time of onset, and duration)

Upon completion of a medical examination or consultation, the company has the right to a written opinion by the attending physician. *However, under no circumstances may the employee's company have access to medical findings or diagnoses that are unrelated to the workplace exposure of that employee.* In order to ensure proper confidentiality between patient and physician regarding non-workplace-related findings or diagnoses, most companies find it most desirable to provide the attending physician with a form that specifically restricts the information provided by the physician to the company to the following:

- results of consultation or examination that are related only to workplace exposure to chemicals
- medical conditions that may place the employee at increased risk when exposed to workplace chemicals
- recommendations for follow-up examinations or tests

If a corporate form for the attending physician is used, that form should also include a clear statement that the physician should not reveal any medical information that is not related to workplace exposure to chemicals. Whatever the form used, the physician should indicate in writing that the employee has been informed by the physician of the results of the consultation or medical examination and any medical condition that may require further examination or treatment.

SAFETY EQUIPMENT AND SUPPLIES

In addition to those considerations of safety that must be consistently applied in the purchase and use of any laboratory equipment (Table 6.2), additional consideration must be given to the type, location, and maintenance requirements of equipment and supplies specifically intended to minimize or manage health and safety risks.

Emergency Eye Washes and Showers

These devices are intended for emergencies in which acute effects are imminent. They must therefore be located for immediate access by people who will likely have difficulty seeing or be otherwise encumbered. A good rule of thumb is that persons should be able to reach an eye wash or shower via an unobstructed route within 3 to 5 sec from the onset of an emergency.

In order to be effective, eye washes must be used continually for 15 min; they should therefore be temperature tempered. Eyewash nozzles should be regularly (e.g., at least monthly) checked for any buildup of grit that can cause physical abrasion of the eye. Emergency showers should be fitted with privacy curtains and bucket-tested at least quarterly to ensure proper water flow.

All personnel must be instructed how to use eye washes and showers both when alone or when aiding a co-worker. This includes detailed instruction (and, ideally, practice) in keeping the eye continually flushed for 15 min, as well as in disrobing while under the shower.

TABLE 6.2   An Example of a Checklist Used for the Prepurchase Evaluation of Laboratory Equipment[a]

1. Structural Material of Equipment • Resistance to shatter • Resistance to corrosion • Resistance to meltdown and ignition • Resistance to chemicals • Longevity • Ease of Cleaning **2. Stress on Laboratory Equipment During Use** • Centrifugal force • Impact • Structural fatigue • Pressure • Surface configuration and finish • Annealing possibly required • Creep (time, temperature and strength relationship) • Temperature (maximum; minimum; duration; cycling) • Corrosion (surface; stress cracking; connecting equipment) **3. Electrical Components** • Capacity (voltage; current) • Grounding requirements • Overload protection • Type (explosion-proof; enclosed; non-sparking) • Emergency shutoff • Lockout capability • Control of static electricity	**4. Mechanical Hazards** • Sharp edges or points • Shields (strength; direction of protection; ease of use; stability; ignitability) • Pressure release (venting mechanism; sensitivity to corrosion; testing requirements) **5. Maintenance** • Lubrication requirements • Inspection requirements • Pressure testing • Accessibility to parts • Standardization of parts **6. Placement of Equipment** • Pedestrian safety • Protrusion of parts • Ease of sample introduction and removal • Adequacy of working space and lighting **7. Operating Instructions** • Clarity • Completeness • Troubleshooting

[a] Adapted from materials provided by Claire G. Erickson.

First Aid Supplies

First aid often becomes confused in the industrial setting with medical treatment. The purpose of first aid is twofold: to keep the patient alive and, where possible, minimize the threat of additional injury until professional medical help becomes available. Toward these objectives, most attention must be directed, in order of priority, to (a) notifying professional medical responders, (b) keeping the patient breathing and preventing profuse loss of blood, and (c) providing a nonthreatening surrounding.

In too many instances, first aid kits contain supplies that are irrelevant to the objectives of first aid and which, in fact, can result in additional health or safety risks. For example, the stocking of first aid kits with such items as lozenges, or inhalants used for everything from stuffy noses to revive employees who have fainted, or allergy medicines or even aspirin should be strongly discouraged. Lozenges not only are useless in stanching profuse bleeding or clearing an obstructed pharynx, they also can absorb ambient atmospheric chemicals and become sources of contamination. Stuffy noses are not the province of first aid; nor is fainting a life-threatening circumstance calling for the inhalation of medicines to which someone may be hypersensitive.

While it is reasonable to include Band-Aids and topical disinfectants to meet the immediate needs of minor cuts and abrasions, first aid supplies should be primarily those to keep (a) injured people breathing and pumping sufficient blood to stay alive until professional medical personnel arrive, and (b) the first aid responder from becoming contaminated while in the process of giving first aid. In most laboratories, such items most reasonably include:

- large pressure bandage, including white towels in sealed plastic
- tourniquet
- shielded guard for mouth-to-mouth resuscitation
- protective gloves
- disinfection materials, adequate for HIV and other bloodborne pathogens

All persons who might be expected to utilize first aid materials must be instructed in the proper use and subsequent disposal of each item.

Spill Containment

A key objective in any health and safety program is the management of spills which, as both a proactive and reactive objective, should be approached from several directions, including:

- Using plastic protected bottles for stock chemicals and hazardous wastes, especially for volumes ≥ 4 liters
- Ensuring that all chemical containers are stored in cabinets fitted with appropriately sized plastic containment trays
- Using plastic containment trays for waste bottles that collect wastes from instrumentation (e.g., HPLC units)
- Using secondary containers for the transport of chemicals to and from as well as within the laboratory
- Fitting all floor drains with secure covers
- Placement of supplies of inert absorbent materials in the immediate areas of potential spills, with particular emphasis given to the speed with which large quantities of the material can be applied to spills

- Disallowing any storage of chemicals in areas that would allow entry of spilled chemicals into wall or floor openings or into conduits for electrical wiring or plumbing
- Installation of hallways mirrors at corridor corners to minimize collisions involving personnel who might be transporting chemicals
- Requiring the use of protective carts for the transport of chemicals in bulk
- Ensuring that bulk stock chemicals in drums are always stored on spill containment platens

Fire Extinguishers

While many fire authorities require the installation of fire extinguishers in laboratories, the CHO should understand that, because of the relatively high nozzle pressure of extinguishers, the stream of the released extinguishing materials may sweep many breakable chemical containers off laboratory benches or cabinets and thereby contribute to explosive and flammable risk, as well as to the risk of toxic fumes generated either through heat or the reactivity of mixed chemicals. Extinguishers should be used in the laboratory only by authorized personnel who have received appropriate training, which should include actual practice. In the absence of an ongoing commitment to such training, the CHO is advised that it is best to focus on laboratory evacuation and to restrict the use of extinguishers to fighting so-called "basket-fires" (i.e., fires that can easily be extinguished with minimal involvement of the overall laboratory space). Of course, the selection of extinguishing materials, including those contained in portable extinguishers or in any automatic fire suppressant system, must be guided by the reactivity (e.g., water reactivity) of laboratory chemicals, and should be undertaken only in strict coordination with fire science professionals.

HEALTH AND SAFETY ANALYSIS OF CHEMICALS

Under the Laboratory Standard, it is expected that each chemical will have been carefully evaluated not only with respect to its meeting a particular operational need, but also with regard to its health and safety implications. As a routine assessment, such a health and safety analysis should be applied to all chemicals, including stock chemicals, chemical by-products produced in chemical or physical reactions, and waste chemicals.

The data considered in the progress of a substance-specific health and safety analysis is usually standardized in a written form or computerized template, which should be approved by the laboratory manager who must coordinate with the CHO for this purpose. They key elements of any comprehensively designed substance-specific health and safety analysis include the following:

- Precise identification of the pure chemical or of the chemical constituents of a mixture, usually the scientific name as well as *Chemical Abstract Service* (CAS) number. The basic rule of thumb is that the identification must allow direct access to the pertinent literature base regarding the health and safety aspects of the substance.
- Those chemical constituents that qualify as "extremely hazardous chemicals" under the laboratory standard. More and more companies also include information on the legal status of each constituent with regard to a range of regulations (e.g., transportation regulations; regulations governing hazardous wastes, etc.).
- The potential acute and chronic health effects of each constituent, including human epidemiological evidence and laboratory studies of animals. The rule of thumb to follow is that the identification of health effects can be based on even a single scientific report—the effects need not be "certified" by governmental authority.
- The potential physical effects of each constituent on living tissue or the whole organism (e.g., fire, explosion, asphyxiation, etc.).
- Special procedures to be implemented for storing or handling the substance in the laboratory.
- Specific health factors that might exclude a laboratory employee from using a particular substance, such as a heart condition or an allergy.
- Specific means for protecting laboratory personnel from exposure to the substance, including procedures, engineering controls, clothing, the use of eye protection devices, protective gloves or aprons, and a respirator. Means for protection should be specified for each step in any laboratory procedure that might result in exposure.
- Special cleanup instructions, including instructions for cleaning glassware and equipment, collecting spills, and disposing of any waste or contaminated materials.
- Emergency procedures and equipment required, usually on the basis of amount of substance spilled, the possible location of an emergency event (e.g., in the chemical store room), or the type of hazard (e.g., toxic gas) presented by an emergency.

REFERENCE INFORMATION

In order to ensure compliance with this standard, the CHO as well as the laboratory employee must have access to reference materials regarding

(a) the health and safety hazards and (b) means for the safe handling, storage, and disposal of those hazardous chemicals that are present in the laboratory. While the MSDSs for chemicals provide such information, the CHO is well advised to understand that reference materials are not to be limited to MSDSs.

Appropriate references, in either printed or computerized format, include such items as toxicological monographs for particular chemicals, catalogs of commercially available safety equipment and supplies, technical and scientific glossaries regarding health and safety related information, and regulatory as well as professional publications regarding prudent practices for laboratories. The CHO might well first consider what informational sources have to be consulted in the progress of conducting the health and safety analysis of chemicals—these are precisely the sources that should be immediately available to laboratory personnel.

CHAPTER 7

LOCKOUT–TAGOUT

BACKGROUND

Known commonly in industry as "LOTO," lockout–tagout is a written *energy control program* that is designed to direct the servicing of machines and equipment in which the unexpected energization or start up, or the release of stored energy could cause physical injury to employees performing maintenance tasks.

In the United States, LOTO regulations (29 CFR 1910.147) specifically exempt so-called "normal production operations"; it focuses on servicing or maintenance operations. However, servicing or maintenance often does take place during normal production operations. In these instances, LOTO regulations also apply whenever an employee is required to:

(a) remove or bypass a guard or other safety device (e.g., to get at a product that has fallen out of its production path and become lodged in some mechanism of the production machine)

(b) place any part of the body into an area on a machine or piece of equipment where work is actually performed upon the material being processed (e.g., capping of bottles along a conveyor filling line), or where an associated danger zone exists during a machine operating cycle (e.g., in vicinity of a heating element).

Also exempted are minor tool changes, machine adjustments, and other minor servicing activities that may take place during normal production operations and that are routine, repetitive, and integral to the use of equipment for production. In such instances, the key consideration is that the worker is appropriately protected while performing these activities by means other than LOTO.

LOTO procedures also do not typically apply to situations where the exposure to a machine's energy hazards, whether active or stored energy, is completely controlled by unplugging the machine's electrical cord—and where the unplugged electrical cord is under the immediate control of the person actually servicing the deactivated machine. By "control" here is meant that the cord cannot be plugged back into a live electrical circuit except with the knowledge of the person performing maintenance. Safety personnel are advised to be extremely cautious in opting for this exemption because there are many circumstances in which a worker may think he has effective control of the electrical plug for a machine under service, but actually does not, or simply makes a mistake and reconnects the plug.

Essentially, the LOTO program focuses on two types of facility personnel: those designated as *authorized personnel*, specifically authorized and trained to perform LOTO on particular machines, and those designated as *affected personnel*, other employees who, though they do not perform LOTO, may be affected by the actual conduct of procedures associated with LOTO.

The overall development of an energy control program is often the responsibility of the plantwide safety officer, regulatory compliance officer, plant engineer, or the director of the human resources department. Sometimes, the supervisor of the maintenance department, or the supervisor of the department in which the actual maintenance service is performed, or the production supervisor is given important if not sole operational authority for its implementation. For purposes of the following text, the safety officer will be assumed to have overall responsibility.

ENERGY CONTROL PROCEDURES

The heart of the energy control program, energy control procedures specify the precise steps to be taken during the servicing of a machine to prevent the accidental release of hazardous energy. Each procedure must be specific to a particular machine; however, in a plant having a number of the same model machines, as is quite common, for example, in a plastic extrusion plant, the same procedure may be used for a group of identical machines.

Prior to developing any energy control procedures, the safety officer must identify all machines or equipment in which the unexpected energizing, start up or release of stored energy could occur and cause injury during servicing or maintenance. Types of energy to be considered include electrical, mechanical (e.g., tension, torsion), hydraulic, pneumatic, chemical, thermal (including cryogenic), and gravitational (e.g., as in an elevated platen that could fall) energy, whether active (as in a live electrical circuit) or potential (as in charged capacitors).

During the identification of machines and equipment to be included in the LOTO program, the safety officer is strongly advised to coordinate directly with plant engineers, machine operators, and maintenance personnel who have practical experience with machinery. Particular attention must be given to the fact that modern industrial equipment typically utilizes different types of energy in both active and potential states.

It is also important that machines and equipment be included in the LOTO program on the basis of their potential for releasing hazardous energy and not on the basis of any other consideration, such as whether or not it must be fully or partially operative for particular types of maintenance, or whether it is serviced by external contractors or by company personnel—both of which issues are specifically addressed by the LOTO regulations.

As shown in Figure 7.1, each energy control procedure must contain the following information:

- Manufacturer's name of the machine or equipment. It is also advisable that the safety officer assign a code number to each machine included in the energy control program to facilitate record keeping. Usually, the list of machine names and associated codes is included as an appendix to the written LOTO program.
- Statement of the specific conditions under which the procedure is to be followed, such as "general maintenance," or "maintenance requiring disassembly," or "annual shutdown and inspection."
- Identification of the various types of active and stored energy, including the amount of each type of energy (e.g., volts, p.s.i., degrees Fahrenheit). Chemical energy hazards should be identified regarding the type of hazard, such as "corrosive," "explosive," or "toxic gas."
- Specific directions for shutting down, isolating, blocking, and securing machine or equipment to control hazardous energy. Basic procedures include using (a) a lock, (b) a warning tag, or (c) restraining devices, such as restraining chains, bars, or (d) any combination of locks, tags, or restraining devices.
- Specific directions for the placement, removal, and transfer of lockout, tagout, or restraining devices, including number and location.
- Specific requirements for testing a machine or the equipment to determine and verify the effectiveness of lockout, tagout, or other energy control measures.
- Any other requirements for ensuring the safety of personnel, including requirements regarding protective clothing and other premaintenance preparations.

With regard to using locks and warning tags, the general rule is to use a lock wherever feasible; where locks are used, warning tags must also be

Global Enterprises, Inc. **Energy Control Procedure**	**Machine Code**	LT 23-C
	Approved on:	July 18, 1996
	Approved by:	Donald Oldman

Manufacturer's Designation of Machine or Equipment

Bag House for Pulverizer Unit

Conditions under Which Lockout/Tagout To Be Implemented

Changing Pulverizer Bags; Maintenance on Unit

Type of Energy	Amount	Lockout Required	Tagout Required	Location
• Electrical Breakers	460 v	Yes	Yes	Circuit

Placement & Removal of Locks & Tags

1. Shut down Pulverizer Panel prior to Lockout/Tagout
2. Attach Lock and Tag to Pulverizer Baghouse Rotary Valve (ALP # 24)
3. Attach Lock and Tag to Breaker for Strip Air Fan (ALP #20)
4. Attach Lock and Tag to Breaker for Vent Fan (ALP #2)
5. Attach Lock and Tag to Breaker for Dehumidification A/C Fan (BC 006)
6. Attach Lock and Tag to Air Line Valve Shut Off on 2nd level above catwalk

Verification of Lockout/Tagout

1. Activate Start Switch to ensure that unit is electrically disconnected
2. Return Start Switch to 'OFF' Position
3. Check Pressure Gauge to ensure proper bleed off of air; do not commence work until gauge reads 'zero'

Other Requirements

1. Wear normal shop uniform
2. Wear routine shop boots

SPECIAL NOTE

You may not commence any maintenance work until you have completed the Log-In Procedure

FIGURE 7.1 Example of an energy control procedure. This procedure contains the basic information required to implement an effective lockout/tagout program. Depending upon the complexity of the procedure, additional information may be provided on the reverse side of this form.

attached in the immediate area of the lock. In many instances, older machines are not equipped by the manufacturer with appropriate lock clasps and the safety officer may therefore opt for the use of warning tags only. However, every reasonable attempt should be made to refit older machines with lock clasps.

All LOTO procedures will be inspected at least annually. The requirements of this inspection are:

1. The inspection will be performed by a person other than an employee who utilizes the procedure.

2. The inspector will identify and correct any deviations or inadequacies observed in the actual implementation of the procedure being inspected. All corrections will be documented and signed by the inspector. Corrections with respect to observed inadequacies of the procedure will be immediately incorporated in the written energy control program. Corrections with respect to employee deviations from a procedure will be appropriately dealt with according to normal personnel procedures, and should also include additional training in the proper use of LOTO procedures.

3. Regarding a procedure that employs locks, the inspection will include a review, between the inspector and each person authorized to perform the LOTO procedure, to ensure that "authorized personnel" understand their responsibilities under that procedure.

4. Regarding a procedure that employs warning tags, the inspection will include a review between the inspector, each person authorized to perform the LOTO procedure, and all other affected employees, to ensure that authorized personnel understand their responsibilities under that procedure.

5. The safety officer will certify that the periodic inspections have been performed. The certification will identify the machine or equipment on which the energy control procedure was utilized, the date of the inspection, the employees included in the inspection, and the person performing the inspection.

LOG-IN PROCEDURE

Documentation regarding the actual conduct of LOTO is important and is most frequently accomplished through the use of a log book. While different companies may have different requirements as to specific log entries, the following is a typical log-in procedure that imparts significant responsibility to a maintenance supervisor, hereinafter referred to as simply "the supervisor."

Prior to any maintenance personnel undertaking the servicing of a machine or equipment, the supervisor will determine if the machine or equipment is included in the LOTO program. If so, each of the following steps must be completed:

1. The supervisor will verify that (a) the employee is specifically authorized in the written energy control program to perform maintenance on the specific machine or equipment and (b) the employee has completed all training requirements associated with the program.

2. The supervisor will provide the authorized employee with (a) the appropriate energy control procedure for the machine or equipment to be repaired and (b) the lockout/tagout hardware identified in the relevant energy control procedure.

3. Both the supervisor and the authorized employee will verify by their signatures in the log book that the proper procedure has been selected, that the proper lockout/tagout hardware has been provided to the employee, and that the employee fully understands the energy control procedure to be followed. The log book will contain the following information:

- the date and time the maintenance or service was initiated and completed
- the name of the equipment or machine serviced
- the LOTO code for the equipment or machine (which is also the code assigned to the written procedure)
- signature of the supervisor and the authorized person(s) performing the service or maintenance

4. Upon completion of the maintenance, it is the responsibility of the authorized employee to return all hardware and the energy control procedure to the supervisor.

LOTO HARDWARE

The basic hardware involved in any energy control program includes three types of devices: (a) an *energy isolating device*, which prevents the transmission or release of energy, such as a circuit breaker, power panel, disconnect switch, and line valve; (b) a *lockout device*, which uses a key or combination to hold an energy isolating device in an active mode (i.e., preventing the flow of energy), and (c) a *tagout device*, which is a prominent tag or sign that can be securely attached to an energy isolating or lockout device and which effectively communicates a warning that the machine or equipment to which it is attached cannot be operated until the tagout device is removed.

LOTO regulations specify the requirements for locks and tags and isolation devices, including requirements pertaining to strength, durability under environmental stress of temperature, humidity and corrosivity, and standardization (in the case of locks) regarding such attributes as color and shape and (in the case of tags), legend and print format. While such regulatory requirements are clear and succinct, there is nonetheless frequent confusion regarding the in-plant management of hardware such as locks and other devices.

For example, in many companies there are often long-standing rules regarding master keys for locks in general. Usually master keys are required and their use is restricted to a particular managerial level. Sometimes, locks may be used daily for a wide variety of purposes, including to secure doors, lockers, and tool boxes. Regardless of such in-plant rules or practices, the safety officer must understand two cardinal rules regarding LOTO that must override all other practices:

> First and foremost, a lock is the primary means whereby an employee guarantees personal protection from a hazard. That lock is therefore to be fitted with only one key, and that key must be in the possession of the employee using it for LOTO. Duplicate or master keys for a LOTO lock must be destroyed.
>
> Second, a lock to be used in the LOTO program must not be used for any other company or personal purpose. Ideally, locks to be used for LOTO should be color coded or otherwise made distinct so that there can be no confusion as to the restricted use of LOTO locks.

While some companies provide personal locks to authorized employees, many provide locks through a centrally located supply, which is best located in the immediate vicinity of the LOTO log book and copies of the energy control procedures. A centrally located supply minimizes the potential use of personally issued locks being used for other than LOTO purposes and also tends to reduce the number of locks that have to be managed. Its colocation with the log book and written procedures also facilitates the practical efficiency of the energy control program.

The concern for ensuring the restricted in-plant use of LOTO locks must extend also to the use of other hardware, including such energy isolation devices as chains used to secure valves, blocks, and wedges used to secure raised machine parts, plug-boots used to isolate electrical cords, and line blind inserts used to block the in-line flow of gas or liquid. Restricted use of items associated with LOTO to only LOTO operations accomplishes two objectives: to ensure that not only will LOTO hardware not become dysfunctional through other use, but also that such items must be specifically selected for their LOTO purpose as opposed to being rigged or otherwise adapted from other functions and, therefore, not likely the most appropriate items to use to ensure safety.

ENERGY ISOLATION

Actual implementation of a LOTO procedure requires the sequential completion of the following seven steps:

1. Notification of affected personnel: Potentially affected employees must be notified of the implementation of a LOTO procedure both prior to its initiation and immediately following its completion. The purpose of this notification is to minimize possible injury to either authorized or affected personnel due to interruption of a portion of the normal production process (e.g., a conveyor line involving staged activities). The supervisor or the authorized personnel must therefore ensure that affected personnel are not only informed of the LOTO procedure, but that they precisely understand how that procedure will affect their work activity.

2. Preparation for shutdown: Before an authorized or affected employee turns off a machine or piece of equipment, the authorized employee must have precise knowledge of the type and magnitude of all relevant active and passive energies associated with the machine or equipment, the safety hazards of the energy to be controlled, and the appropriate method and means for controlling the hazardous energy. The proper way of ensuring that authorized personnel have this knowledge is to require they have the written LOTO procedure in their possession at the machine or equipment being serviced.

3. Machine or equipment shutdown: Shutdown will be accomplished precisely as contained in the written LOTO procedure. Should the authorized person become aware of any necessary deviation from printed directions in the LOTO procedure, that person must immediately abort that procedure and consult the maintenance supervisor to resolve the discrepancy. Under no circumstances will authorized personnel proceed except in a manner specifically dictated by the written directions of the LOTO procedure.

4. Isolation of machine or equipment: The authorized person must position and utilize all energy isolating devices as specified in the written LOTO procedure. Under no circumstances will any substitute device be made (e.g., using a rope instead of a specified chain to secure the closed position of a valve) or any specified device be ignored.

5. Attachment of lockout or tagout devices: Lockout or tagout devices will be affixed to each energy isolating device only by authorized employees. Lockout devices will be affixed in such a manner that they will hold the energy isolating device in the "safe" position (i.e., preventing the flow of energy). Tagout devices will be affixed in such a manner that they will clearly indicate that the operation or movement of energy isolating devices from the safe position is prohibited. Where only tagout devices are used with those energy isolating devices that have the capability of being locked, the tag will

be fastened at the same point at which a lock would have been attached. Where a tag cannot be affixed directly to the energy isolating device, the tag will be located as close as safely possible to the device, in a position that will be immediately obvious to anyone attempting to operate the device.

6. Control of stored energy: Following the application of lockout or tagout devices to energy isolating devices and in precise conformity with directions included in the written LOTO procedure, all potentially hazardous stored or residual energy will be relieved, disconnected, restrained, or otherwise rendered safe. If there is any possibility of a reaccumulation of stored energy to a hazardous level, verification of isolation (see below) will be continued until the servicing or maintenance is completed, or until the possibility of such accumulation no longer exists.

7. Verification of isolation: Prior to starting work on machines or equipment that have been locked or tagged out, the authorized employee will verify that isolation and deenergization of the machine or equipment have been actually accomplished. Verification procedures included in the written LOTO procedure must be precisely followed and under no circumstance will be altered or aborted.

RELEASE FROM LOCKOUT OR TAGOUT

Before lockout or tagout devices are removed and energy is restored to the machine or equipment, authorized personnel must inspect the work area to ensure that nonessential items have been removed and that machine or equipment components are operationally intact. Before machines or equipment are energized, affected employees will be notified that the lockout or tagout procedure is completed, and the work area will be examined to ensure that all employees have been safety positioned for machine or equipment start up.

Each lockout or tagout device must be removed from each energy isolating mechanism only by the employee who applied that device. This requirement calls for two different procedures, depending upon whether the employee is unavailable because of a change in work-shifts or is otherwise unavailable (e.g., due to a personal emergency).

In the case of a shift-change, it is the responsibility of the authorized employee who initiates the LOTO procedure for a particular machine or equipment to transfer lockout or tagout devices between off-going and on-coming employees. The initiating authorized employee responsible for this transfer will notify the supervisor that the transfer has been accomplished. The oncoming authorized employee is responsible for completing the log-in procedure and all subsequent procedures in the energy control program.

When the authorized employee who applied the lockout or tagout device is otherwise not available to remove it, that device may be removed (in the case of locks, by cutting) under the direction of the supervisor, provided that the following steps are taken:

- The supervisor verifies that the authorized employee who applied the device is not available,
- All reasonable efforts are made to contact and inform the authorized employee that the lockout or tagout device is to be removed by another person, and
- There is full assurance that the authorized employee will be informed of the removal of the device before the employee resumes work at the facility.

The supervisor is well advised to document all actions taken in the progress of completing the above steps.

SPECIAL PROCEDURES

Given the diversity and complexity of industrial processes, any practical energy control program must make provision for special circumstances regarding the operational requirements of specific machinery and equipment, company practices regarding contractors, and the use of maintenance crews.

Testing or Adjustment of Machines and Equipment

The servicing of many types of machines and equipment often requires periodic activation of machinery in order to test or adjust performance. This requirement is often mistakenly used to preclude inclusion of a particular machine in the formal energy control program. The safety officer must understand that a machine becomes subject to LOTO regulations solely on the basis of the potential for a sudden release of hazardous energy that can injure personnel—not on the basis of any operational requirement of the machine.

Periodic reactivation of machines and equipment during servicing is clearly addressed by LOTO regulations, including reactivation for the purposes of testing, positioning, or adjusting machine and equipment performance. The basic rules governing this type of operation are as follows:

1. Prior to reactivation, clear the machine or equipment of tools and other maintenance-related materials to ensure that machine or equipment operations are functionally unobstructed.

2. Ensure that all employees in the general area are safety positioned.
3. Remove relevant lockout, tagout, and energy isolating devices in accordance with written LOTO procedures.
4. Reenergize machine, equipment, or component and complete testing, adjustment, and/or repositioning of the machine or equipment.
5. Deenergize all systems and reapply energy control measures in accordance with written LOTO procedures and continue with servicing or maintenance.

Contractors

The historic reliance upon the professional judgment of contractors as to how they accomplish what they are paid to do is no longer (if it ever was) tenable. Contractors not only present a risk to themselves, but also to the employees of the company that hires them. In order to manage the health and safety risks of both company employees and contractor personnel, as well as the legal liabilities potentially related to the activities of contractors, the safety officer must ensure contractor compliance with LOTO regulations.

Should a contractor service any machine or equipment that is included in a company's LOTO program, the minimal requirement is that the safety officer and the contractor inform each other of their respective procedures. Under no circumstances should a contractor be allowed to service a machine or equipment included in the company's LOTO program without implementing a LOTO procedure.

The safety officer is also best advised that a contractor's procedure for a specific machine or equipment should be at least as stringent as the company's LOTO procedure. Also, in the case where the contractor uses his own LOTO procedure, the company safety officer should maintain a copy of the contractor's procedure. Finally, the safety officer should ensure (a) that company personnel fully understand and comply with any restrictions and prohibitions imposed by the contractor's energy control procedures and (b) that under no circumstance shall company personnel or contractor personnel remove each others' energy isolation, locking, or tagging devices.

Group Lockout or Tagout

Often the maintenance or servicing of a machine or equipment requires the effort of two or more persons. In such instances, so-called "group lockout and tagout procedures" are required in order to provide the work crew a level of protection equivalent to that provided by a personal lockout or tagout device. Group lockout and tagout devices are to be used in accordance with the following requirements:

1. Primary responsibility is vested in an authorized employee for a number of employees working under the protection of a group lockout or tagout device; this responsibility is inclusive of all requirements regarding log-in, the procurement of copies of written LOTO procedures and hardware, and the conduct of LOTO procedures;

2. The authorized employee having primary responsibility can directly determine the status of individual group members with regard to potential exposure to hazardous energy;

3. When more than one group is involved, assignment of overall job-associated lockout or tagout responsibility is assigned to an authorized employee specifically designated to coordinate affected workers and to ensure continuity of worker protection; and

4. Each authorized employee will affix a personal lockout or tagout device to the group lockout device, group lockbox, or comparable mechanism and, having completed his own service or maintenance function, will personally remove his own lockout or tagout devices. Where a group tagout device is used, such as a single tag that contains the name of each member of the group, the employee who has completed his task will remove his name from the group tag.

TRAINING AND COMMUNICATION

The LOTO training program must ensure that the purpose and function of the energy control program are understood by authorized and affected employees and that the knowledge and skills required for the safe application, use, and removal of energy controls are effectively translated into job performance. Specific requirements include:

1. Each authorized employee will receive training in the recognition of applicable hazardous energy sources, the type and magnitude of the hazardous energy, and the methods and physical means necessary to isolate and control hazardous energy.

2. Each affected employee will be instructed in the purpose and use of energy control procedures.

3. All other employees whose work operations are in an area where energy control procedures are utilized will be instructed about the purpose of the procedure and any prohibitions regarding attempts to restart or re-energize machines or equipment that are locked or tagged out.

4. When only tagout procedures are used, employees will be trained in the following limitations of tags:

- Tags are essentially warning devices affixed to energy isolating devices and do not provide the physical restraints on those devices provided by a lock.
- When a tag is attached to an energy isolating device, it is not to be removed without authorization by the person responsible for it, and it is never to be bypassed, ignored, or otherwise defeated.
- Tags must be legible and understandable by all authorized employees, affected employees, and all other employees (and contractors) whose work operations are in the general area.
- Tags may evoke a false sense of security, and their meaning needs to be understood as part of the overall energy control program.
- Tags must be securely attached to energy isolating devices so they cannot be inadvertently or accidentally detached during use; under no circumstances is any employee to tamper with an attached tag.

5. Retraining of personnel must be conducted whenever a periodic inspection reveals, or the supervisor or safety officer has reason to believe, that there are deviations from or inadequacies in the employee's knowledge or use of energy control procedures.

CHAPTER 8

CONFINED SPACE ENTRY AND HOTWORK

BACKGROUND

The hazards associated with confined space entry (CSE) and with hotwork (HW) are the focus of two distinct sets of American regulations (29 CFR 1910.146 and 29 CFR 1910.252, respectively). However, both sets of regulations involve the use of in-plant permits and it is therefore generally more efficient to combine company policies regarding these two issues in a single compliance document.

Essentially, a confined space (a) has limited openings for human entry and exit (i.e., lack of standard doors associated with a typical room) and (b) may present entering personnel with safety hazards due to gases, vapors, or other physical hazards. Typical examples of confined spaces include (but are certainly not limited to) manholes, tunnels, wells, cold storage lockers, tanks, sewers, subcellars, ship holds, vaults, and silos. Any of these confined spaces may involve risk due to a variety of circumstances, such as the accumulation of toxic or explosive fumes, the displacement of breathable air (i.e., asphyxiation), and the presence of physical threats such as electrical discharge (e.g., in an underground electrical transformer vault) or mechanical injury (e.g., entanglement in a stirring mechanism within a large reactor vessel or engulfment by materials stored in a silo).

While different types of confined spaces present different types of safety hazards, all confined spaces typically share a common feature—escape and rescue are difficult. Most deaths associated with confined spaces involve would-be rescuers. In particular instances, several or even dozens of persons attempting the rescue of even a single person from a confined space may be seriously injured if not killed outright.

Hotwork is defined as any work that results in the generation of an open flame, or spark, or sufficient heat to cause fire or explosion, including such commonly performed work as welding, grinding, drilling, and cutting. Hotwork performed by a single person in an isolated location can result in the generation of fire, explosion, and toxic fumes that can affect large numbers of people in distant locations, including the surrounding community.

While permits regarding work in confined spaces and hotwork are typically generated within a company for company use, they must be viewed (as must any written industrial health or safety program) essentially as contracts between the company, its employees, and the community at large. As with any contract, a confined space or hotwork permit is a binding agreement that the company will perform or refrain from undertaking specific actions and activities. Today, the measure of the adequacy of actions and activities directed toward human health and safety objectives is increasingly what is often referred to as "state-of-art," the best possible actions that can be taken for a given situation.

In most companies, overall responsibility for confined space entry and hotwork procedures is usually given to the maintenance supervisor or the corporate safety officer, although it is not uncommon in relatively small companies to assign this responsibility to production personnel. In the following text, it is assumed that the safety officer has prime responsibility.

IDENTIFICATION OF CONFINED SPACES AND HAZARDS

The basis of any CSE program is a comprehensive audit of the facility (including both grounds and buildings) to identify specific confined spaces and the various hazards that may be associated with each. This identification should be made only on the basis of limitations on access and regress and potential hazards, the latter usually being due to poor ventilation, but also possibly due to such factors as potential engulfment (as in a collapse of ditched walls). Identification of confined spaces should not be influenced by other considerations, such as a work area being restricted to only contractor personnel, or an area that is present on company property but is not used (e.g., a vacant subcellar or long abandoned subground vault).

Primary hazards to be examined with respect to each confined space include:

- Oxygen deficiency or overabundance
- Flammable gas or vapor
- Toxic gas or vapor
- Engulfment
- Mechanical hazard

TABLE 8.1   Vapor Density and Flashpoint Values for Some Common Organic Solvents

Solvent	Vapor density[a]	Flashpoint (°F)[b]
Methanol	1.1	65
Ethanol	1.6	57
Acetone	2.0	0
Isopropanol	2.1	70
Butanol	2.5	52
Tetrahydrofuran	2.5	1
Petroleum ether	2.5	0
Benzene	2.8	12
Furfural	3.3	140
Isopropyl ether	3.5	15
Heptane	3.5	30
n-Butyl ether	4.5	70

Air = 1

[a] Vapor density (vd) relative to air, where vd (air) = 1. *Weight to unit volume*
[b] Flashpoint (*lowest temperature at which vapor is flammable*) on basis of open or closed cup test; values rounded off to nearest integer.

Heavier then air will collect low or underground.

- Electrical shock
- Skin hazard
- Eye hazard

Such hazards are not mutually exclusive and, in fact, may jointly contribute to or even synergistically interact to multiply the safety risk of a particular confined space. For example, oxygen deficiency (i.e., <19.5% of air by volume) may occur in a confined space due to excessive microbial decomposition of organic materials (as in sewage). Decomposition (*mineralization*) is a process that can also produce toxic gases such as hydrogen sulfide, flammable gases such as methane, and asphyxiants such as carbon dioxide. Oxygen deficiency may also occur due to displacement of air by heavier vapors, including many toxic and flammable vapors that have vapor densities higher than air (Table 8.1). A confined space in which flammable vapors can displace air and which also contains potential sources of ignition (e.g., electrical and nonsparking manual tools, electrical circuits) obviously presents high risk not only to workers within that space, but also to company personnel and the general public in the immediate vicinity.

Not only do confined spaces vary greatly with regard to types of hazards and the cause of those hazards, but also in terms of degree or, more technically, actual risk. While both a silo and a silo substage (which accommodates the conical, continual feed portion of the silo) may present an engulfment hazard, the risk of engulfment varies greatly between them. In the case of the silo itself, there is a constant risk due to stored materials. In the substage, there is a negligible risk because its realization would require actual structural collapse which, although possible, is highly improbable within the engineered lifetime of the structure.

Because of the large variability of risks among confined spaces, some legal authorities allow for the designation of confined spaces as "permit-requiring" or "non-permit-requiring" confined spaces in accordance with high-risk and low-risk criteria. Where legally permitted, many companies opt for this distinction because non-permit-requiring confined spaces imply less costly management or compliance effort. However, such judgments should always be evaluated from a projected perspective of "postincident hindsight"—what might appear to be not only legal but also eminently logical as well as a real economic saving prior to an actual safety incident most often actually proves to be the precise source of that significant economic and legal anxiety that is almost certain to be experienced after an incident.

The proactive approach for effective management of both human safety and corporate liability is to declare all confined spaces as permit-requiring and to deal with variations in risks among confined spaces in terms of different substantive requirements for different confined spaces. For example, having made the judgment that all confined spaces within company jurisdiction should be treated as permit-requiring confined spaces, a company will typically be acting well within the constraints of regulatory objectives and requirements to distinguish among permit-requiring confined spaces as follows:

- Class I (lowest risk): those confined spaces where the atmosphere cannot develop a dangerous air contaminant or oxygen deficiency or overabundance and where all known sources of hazards are positively controlled
- Class II (intermediate risk): those confined spaces where an atmosphere free of dangerous air contamination and of any oxygen deficiency or overabundance is verified through documented testing prior to entry and throughout the period of confined space work
- Class III (highest risk): those confined spaces where the presence of dangerous air contamination, oxygen deficiency or overabundance, or other safety hazard cannot be positively controlled under all foreseeable circumstances

It must be emphasized that the above classes (or typology) are not used here as classes having any regulatory basis; they are included only by way of example. The adequacy of such a typology of permit-requiring confined spaces depends, of course, on the specifically mandated procedures to be implemented for each type.

CSE PROCEDURES AND PERMITS

CSE procedures typically focus on three groups of personnel: *authorized entrants*, personnel specifically authorized to enter and work within confined spaces; *authorized attendants*; personnel required to provide immediate safety assistance to authorized entrants but who must remain outside of the confined space; and the *rescue team*, which, in the event of an emergency involving a worker within a confined space, must attempt to rescue that worker.

CSE procedures pertinent to each confined space must include specific information and requirements regarding:

- Nature of hazards associated with the CSE
- Preparation that authorized entrants, attendants, and rescue team members must make prior to initiated work in the CSE
- Protective clothing and equipment required for working in the CSE

Ultimately, information and requirements regarding the conduct of work in a particular confined space are summarized in the form of a permit, such as the one depicted in Figure 8.1, which, in addition to the above information, provides space for (a) listing the names of persons who are authorized to serve as entrants and attendants, (b) recording any monitoring requirements, and (c) certification by a supervisor.

Where a company uses typology of confined spaces on the basis of degree of risk, such as the above typology that includes three distinct classes, the same format of permit is usually used for each type of confined space, with different entries reflecting the differences in degree of risk. The reverse side of the permit is also frequently used to provide additional or clarifying information, such as a glossary of terms, specific procedures for ventilating a particular confined space, company or manufacturers' codes for specific protective equipment, and data related to ambient monitoring.

Whatever the class of permit (i.e., Class I, II, or III or some other typology regarding degree of risk), permits must be dated. Most often, permits for confined spaces that present very limited and controllable risk are attached to the confined space to which they pertain and are valid for 1 year from the date of issue. This approach allows work to be conducted in such a confined space without implementing the following log-in procedure. All other permits (e.g., Class II and Class III) must be dated at the time work is initiated and completed and require authorized personnel and the appropriate supervisor to complete the log-in procedure.

Global Enterprises, Inc. — Confined Space Entry Permit

Confined Space Identification	Monorail Rinse Modules	Entry Procedure	II

(handwritten marginal notes: "Very Dangerous.", "must should Training", "Demostrate Training Once a year")

Today's Date [blank] **Permit Expiration** July 26, 1996

Description of Work [blank]

Nature of Hazard
- ☐ Oxygen deficiency
- ☐ Oxygen overabudance
- ☑ Toxic Gas or Vapor
- ☐ Mechanical Hazard
- ☐ Electrical Shock
- ☑ Skin Hazard
- ☑ Eye Hazard
- ☐ Engulfment
- Other [blank]

Authorized Entrants
[blank]

Authorized Attendants
[blank]

Preparation
- ☑ Notify affected department
- ☑ Complete Lockout-Tagout
- ☐ Clean, drain, wash & purge
- ☐ Complete radio test Ventilate
- ☑ Rescue team available Implement monitoring
- ☐ Attach Hotwork Permit
- ☑ Review procedures & hazards
- ☐ Other [blank]

Safety Clothing & Equipment
- ☐ Respirator [blank]
- ☑ Communication — Keep visual and oral
- ☐ Rescue Equipment [blank]
- ☐ Lifeline [blank]
- ☐ Safety Harness [blank]
- ☑ Protective Clothing — Safety shoes, boots,
- ☑ Eye Protection — Goggles
- ☐ Hearing Protection [blank]
- ☑ Other — Nitrile boots & gloves and goggles for rinse stages 1 & 2 only; safety glasses for other rinse stages

	Parameter	Limit	Time	Reading	Time	Reading
☐	Oxygen (minimum)	19.5 %				
☐	Oxygen (maximum)	22.0 %				
☐	Flammability	10%LEL				
☐	Hydrogen Sulfide	10 ppm				
☐	Carbon Monoxide	50 ppm				
☐	Heat	75° F				
☐	Toxic (specify)					
☐	Other (specify)					

FIGURE 8.1 Example of a confined space permit. In this case, the permit is issued by the maintenance manager. Shaded portions are to be filled in by workers undertaking the work. Black squares indicate specific information and requirements that pertain to the identified confined space. Such a permit will often contain an authorization block to be signed by the person who issues the permit. Upon completion of the work assignment, the workers return the completed permit to the maintenance manager (or other corporate authority).

Log-in Procedure

The log-in procedure is an essential managerial tool for ensuring that authorized personnel have in their personnel possession all materials required to work safely in a confined space, including the CSE permit and all materials and information prescribed by the permit. It also provides the means for documenting CSE and is therefore an essential data base for meeting various reporting needs under pertinent regulations. With the possible exception of work to be undertaken in a confined space specifically identified as requiring only an annual and posted permit, no work in confined space should be undertaken without completion of the log-in procedure.

The safety officer is best advised to establish a bound notebook in which handwritten entries document the log-in process. Appropriate column headings include:

- Date and time when an authorized employee begins the log-in procedure
- Name of initiating authorized employee
- Identification (name or code) of specific confined space
- Description of proposed work
- Date and time when work is begun
- Date and time when work is actually completed
- Signature of authorized employee performing log-in
- Signature of supervisor

It is critical that it be clearly understood that, by their signatures, the authorized employee and the supervisor in fact certify the following:

1. That he or she is in fact listed as an authorized employee for the indicated confined space
2. That the authorized employee has obtained the correct permit for the indicated confined space as well as all hardware, materials, and information specified in that permit
3. That all required entries in the permit (e.g., list of authorized entrants and attendants) have been properly completed
4. That the authorized employee understands how to implement all procedures identified in the permit
5. That the authorized employee has completed all necessary preparations (including those required by other regulations, such as lockout–tagout regulations) specified in the permit

Upon completion of the indicated work, the CSE permit must be returned to the supervisor, who should review the permit to ensure proper completion of any required entries (e.g., monitoring data) made during the progress of work. Completed permits should be retained by the corporate safety officer in permanent health and safety files.

Practical Management of Permits

In order to facilitate and control the proper use of CSE permits, most companies find it practical for the maintenance supervisor (or safety officer) to maintain a master set of permits as well as working copies at a central location, along with the log-in book, and any other hardware, protective devices, or materials related to CSE. Master sets of permits, which are usually plasticized for protection and contained in a notebook, are basically used as standard references and cannot be altered except through regularly scheduled reviews of corporate CSE policies. Working copies of each permit are those issued to authorized employees on a per-entry basis, with entries being written in as required (e.g., names of personnel) and completed copies being entered into the company's permanent health and safety records.

In cases where annual permits are issued for least hazardous confined spaces (e.g., Class I, as discussed above), the annual permit posted on the relevant confined space is identical to the supervisor's master copy, except that it includes a specific expiration date. Upon renewal, the expired permit is maintained in the safety officer's records of CSE activity.

Contractors

As with Lockout–Tagout procedures (Chapter 7), corporate CSE permits should serve as minimal requirements for all company contractors. Where the contractor chooses to implement additional procedures, the safety officer should maintain a written copy of those procedures and append them to normal in-house documentation of CSE activity. It is prudent that the safety officer require all contractors who perform work in confined spaces to complete the corporate log-in procedure for CSE, with appropriate reference to any contractor-amended corporate permit.

PERFORMANCE TRAINING OF CSE PERSONNEL

The training of personnel having CSE responsibilities must be directly relevant to the job-related responsibilities of authorized entrants, authorized attendants, and the rescue team. As with all other regulated aspects of workplace health and safety, personnel training that consists primarily of the passive watching of training films or reading printed materials is not relevant, is not meaningful, and is not sufficient. Actual job performance is the only useful measure of any health and safety training program.

Entrants

Personnel who are authorized to serve as CSE entrants must be able to demonstrate their ability to:

1. Determine if they are specifically authorized under CSE regulations to undertake work in any particular confined space,

2. Recognize and describe the range of hazards presented by each confined space in which they are authorized to work,

3. Recognize the signs and symptoms of potential hazardous exposures and describe the possible health and safety consequences of each type of exposure,

4. Implement the appropriate response to signs and symptoms of hazardous exposure,

5. Properly utilize and maintain all protective clothing and equipment, monitoring devices, communication equipment, and any other instrumentation, equipment, or materials specified in a CSE permit, and

6. Recognize the need and implement procedures for safe evacuation from a confined space.

Attendants

Having ultimate responsibility as both the immediate auditor of the health and safety condition of CSE entrants and the *first responder* to an actual CSE emergency, attendants must, under all circumstances, remain stationed outside the permitted space but also maintain constant awareness of actual and developing conditions that may affect the health and safety of workers within that space. Training that is commensurate with these responsibilities should therefore demonstrate the attendant's ability to:

1. Test, operate, and maintain any communication device used to maintain communication with workers within the confined space as well as with any other personnel (e.g., safety officer, supervisors, CSE rescue team) who may be immediately required in the event of a CSE emergency,

2. Test, operate, and maintain any device used to monitor the ambient atmosphere of the confined space or any other condition within the confined space (e.g., temperature, depth of water) that may present a health or safety risk,

3. Test, operate, and maintain any item that is integral to any system employed for the retrieval of personnel within a confined space, including manual or motor-assisted winches, tripods, or body lines,

4. Test, operate, and maintain any warning or alarm system associated with CSE conditions or the health conditions of workers in the confined space,

5. Recognize signs and symptoms of hazardous exposures of workers in the confined space, including developing health symptoms (e.g., worker's becoming disoriented) and behavioral changes (failure of workers to meet voice check schedule),

6. Implement appropriate response to developing conditions within the confined space or the plant (e.g., plant power outage or fire), including initiating confined space evacuation procedures and alerting the rescue team.

Rescue Team

Few companies devote the significant resources in time, money, expertise, and personnel that are realistically commensurate with the actual requirements of rapid, effective, and safe emergency rescue under any circumstance. In fact, even with a willingness to make a significant investment toward this objective, it is highly questionable whether any but a very few companies can realistically be expected to achieve more than what may best be described as a "reasonably good effort"—an effort that, despite even the best of intent, is often limited by factors beyond a company's actual control. The fact that most deaths and injuries associated with CSE involve wouldbe rescuers might well suggest that rescue teams too often attempt to do too much with too little, whether it be too little knowledge, too little experience, too little means or, in many instances, too little luck. The rescue of an endangered human is not always the result of the high daring and bravery but also, especially in modern industry, itself a high art and science that requires essentially the constant practice of professionally tested acumen.

Recognizing the manifold complexity and consequences of mounting a rescue effort, any company is well advised to establish corporate rescue policy only after considering:

1. How to minimize the safety and health risk of those who must perform the rescue effort,

2. How best to ensure that the rescue effort does not contribute to the expansion of an ongoing emergency or develop into a new emergency, with increasing threat to other employees and the general public, and

3. How best to coordinate in-plant and external, professional rescue services to successfully manage the rescue effort.

In its assessment of alternative strategies, the company should make every effort to elicit the recommendations and consultation of external authorities (e.g., fire department, ambulance, and other emergency medical services and local and other governmental agencies), including other companies having similar needs and concerns.

While the rescue effort is an integral component of any *emergency response program* and, as such, is considered in greater detail in Chapter 13, it is reasonable to suggest that the typical in-plant rescue team devoted to CSE should be expected to be highly constrained regarding allowed activities.

For example, it is very common for companies to insist that no member of an in-plant rescue team shall, under any circumstance, enter a confined space for the purpose of rescue. This policy is generally adopted because of the company's clear (and eminently sensible and responsible) recognition that rescue team members, being full-time production personnel and only periodic emergency personnel, cannot maintain a high level of preparedness, regardless of any training effort, and that they themselves are therefore at high risk in any emergency requiring them to attempt to rescue a co-worker.

Where the effort of the rescue team is restricted to the outside of a confined space, the primary objectives of the rescue team are: (a) to utilize external retrieval systems (e.g., winched life-line) to effect the release of personnel from the confined space, (b) to provide CPR or other first aid to extracted personnel, and (c) to take whatever other steps may be necessary to lessen the degree of hazard within the confined space (e.g., implementing remote shutoff of sources of hazard) or maintain the life of entrapped personnel (e.g., providing breathable air) until external, professional assistance arrives on scene.

Because in-plant rescue teams generally operate under such a restriction on their access to a confined space, the training required for the rescue team is different from what it would be if entry were permitted. The following performance skills therefore may or may not apply to a specific team, depending upon this or other policy constraints:

1. Test, operate, and maintain any item that is integral to a system employed for the retrieval of personnel within a confined space, including communication devices and manual or motor assisted winches, tripods, or body lines,

2. Test, operate, and maintain any item of protective clothing, equipment, or device to be used during the retrieval of personnel from a confined space, including ambient and personal monitoring devices and alarms,

3. Perform CPR or any other required first aid procedure, and

4. Perform decontamination of any rescue equipment or materials that might become exposed to hazardous chemicals, including personal protective clothing.

Generally, CSE regulations require that at least one member of the rescue team maintain certification in CPR and basic first-aid, and that the rescue team practice confined space rescues at least annually, using mannequins or actual personnel.

Supervisors of Entrants and Attendants

Often overlooked in training programs devoted to CSE are the supervisors of entrants and attendants, who often play key oversight and quality control roles. The safety officer should ensure that these supervisors receive performance-based training that is commensurate with their CSE responsibilities. Depending upon company policy, these might include their responsibility to:

1. Determine that the entry permit used by authorized entrants does contain the requisite information before authorizing or allowing entry,

2. Determine that the necessary procedures, practices and equipment for safe entry are operational before allowing entry,

3. Determine, at appropriate intervals, that entry operations remain consistent with the terms of the entry permit,

4. Cancel the entry authorization and terminate entry whenever acceptable entry conditions become unacceptable,

5. Ensure that all confined space permits contain or reference, as necessary, appropriate procedures and forms (e.g., lockout–tagout procedures) required by written corporate policies regarding relevant regulations,

6. Take appropriate measures to remove unauthorized personnel who are in or near areas involving confined space operations, and

7. Ensure that contractors conform precisely with all confined space permit requirements.

HOTWORK PROCEDURES AND PERMITS

Just as CSE procedures may be based on a typology of risks associated with the different hazards of different confined spaces, so hotwork procedures may be based on a typology or risks associated with fire and explosion. One such typology for hotwork is as follows:

- Class A (low risk): hotwork conducted where flammables or combustibles are not present in the immediate area (i.e., within 35 feet of the hotwork) and where the hotwork does not involve open flames (e.g., drilling)

- Class B (high risk): hotwork conducted where flammables or combustibles are commonly used or stored and where the hotwork involves open flames or sparks

Examples of hotwork permits (Classes A and B) are included in Figures 8.2 and 8.3. Each of these permits requires the supervisor of the persons performing the work to complete the checklist and to verify by signature that (a) he has personally examined the area where the work is to be performed and (b) the appropriate precautions have been taken. In many cases, the relevant supervisor is the maintenance supervisor. However, in some companies the safety officer (especially when the hotwork is performed by a contractor) or the production supervisor is given this responsibility.

The signed hotwork permit must be prominently displayed in the immediate area of the work being performed. Upon completion of the work, the permit is returned to the authorizing supervisor and entered into permanent corporate health and safety records.

Commonly accepted prudent practices regarding fire safety, which are typically included as regulatory requirements for the conduct of hotwork (e.g., 29 CFR 1910.252), should be meticulously followed by the supervisor prior to authorizing the initiation of hotwork. Such practices and requirements include the following:

1. All movable fire hazards in the vicinity of the work will be removed. Where fire hazards cannot be removed, guards and barriers will be used to confine heat, sparks, and slag, and to protect immovable fire hazards.

2. Wherever there are floor openings or cracks in the flooring that cannot be closed, precautions will be taken so that no readily combustible materials on the floor below will be exposed to sparks that might drop through the floor. The same precautions will be observed with regard to cracks or holes in walls, open doorways, and open or broken windows.

3. Suitable fire extinguishing equipment will be maintained in a state of readiness for instant use.

4. Fire watchers will be required whenever welding or cutting is performed in locations where other than a minor fire might develop or any of the following conditions exist:

- there is appreciable combustible material (in building construction or contents) closer than 35 feet to the point of operation
- appreciable combustibles are more than 35 feet away but are easily ignited by sparks
- wall or floor openings within a 35-foot radius expose combustible material in adjacent areas, including spaces in walls or floors

Global Enterprises, Inc.   **Hotwork Permit: Class A**

Hot Work Performed by:
☐ Global, Inc.
☐ Contractor

Date

Name

Location of Work

Person(s)

Permit Expiration
Date: ____ Time: ____

NA	Required	**Precautions**
☐	☐	Personnel have reviewed Global Confined Space Entry and Hot Work Program
☐	☐	Available sprinklers, hose streams and extinguishers are operational
☐	☐	Flammable liquids, dust, lint and oily deposits within 35 feet of the work area have been removed
☐	☐	There is no explosive atmosphere in the work area
☐	☐	Floors within 35 feet have been swept clean; other combustibles have been removed where possible
☐	☐	Enclosed equipment has been cleaned of all combustibles
☐	☐	Containers have been purged of flammable liquids or vapors
☐	☐	Fire watch will be provided during work (including any breaks) and for 30 minutes after work is completed

Other Necessary Precautions

I verify that the above location has been examined and that the precautions checked on this permit have been taken and hereby authorize the work to proceed

Supervisor's Signature ____   Date ____

FIGURE 8.2 Example of a hotwork permit. This particular permit (Class A; see text), is a less stringent permit for use where the work will not involve open flame or occur in the immediate vicinity of flammable liquids or vapors. Upon issuing the permit, the supervisor checks off the appropriate squares to specify requirements for the particular work and location.

Global Enterprises, Inc.   Hotwork Permit: Class B

Hot Work Performed by:

☐ Global, Inc.

Date

☐ Contractor   Name

Location of Work

Person(s)

Permit Expiration

Date: Time:

General Requirements

☐ Personnel have reviewed Global Confined space and Hot Work Program

☐ Available sprinklers, hose stems and extinguishers are operational

☐ Hotwork equipment is in good repair

Requirements within 35 ft of Work

☐ Flammable liquids, dust, lint and oily deposits have been removed

☐ Explosive atmosphere in area has been eliminated

☐ Floors swept clean; combustible floors wet down, covered with damp sand or fire-resistive sheets

☐ Other combustibles have been removed where possible; otherwise protected with fire-resistive tarpaulins or metal shields

☐ Wall and floor openings covered; fire-resistive tarpaulins suspended beneath

Work on Walls/Ceilings

☐ Construction is noncombustible and without combustible covering or insulation

☐ Combustibles on other side of walls moved away

Work on Enclosed Equipment

☐ Enclosed equipment cleaned of all combustibles

☐ Containers purged of flammable liquids and vapors

Fire Watch

☐ Fire watch will be provided during and for 60 minutes after work, including any breaks

☐ Fire watch is provided with suitable extinguishers/charged hose and is appropriately trained

☐ Monitor Hotwork area for 4 hours after job is completed

Other Necessary Precautions

I verify that the above location has been examined and that the precautions checked on this permit have been taken and hereby authorize the work to proceed

Supervisor's Signature   Date

FIGURE 8.3 Class B permit (see text) for use where the work will involve open flames or take place where flammable liquids or vapors are present. Procedures for issuing this permit are the same as those for the Class A permit (Figure 8.2).

- combustible materials are adjacent to the opposite side of metal partitions, walls, ceilings, or roofs and are likely to be ignited by conduction or radiation.

5. Fire watchers will have fire extinguishing equipment readily available and be trained in its use. They will be familiar with facilities for sounding an alarm in the event of a fire. They will watch for fires in all exposed areas, try to extinguish them only when obviously within the capacity of the equipment available, or otherwise sound the alarm. A fire watch will be maintained for at least one-half hour after completion of welding or cutting operations to detect and extinguish possible smoldering fires.

6. Where combustible materials are on the floor, the floor will be swept clean for a radius of 35 feet. Combustible floors will be kept wet, covered with damp sand, or protected with fire-resistant shields. Where floors have been wet down, personnel operating arc welding or cutting equipment will be protected from possible shock.

7. Cutting or welding will not be permitted in (a) areas not authorized by a hotwork permit, (b) in a sprinklered building while such protection is impaired, (c) in the presence of explosive atmospheres that may develop inside uncleaned or improperly prepared tanks or equipment that have previously contained such materials or that may develop in areas with an accumulation of combustible dusts, or (d) in areas near the storage of large quantities of exposed, readily ignitable materials.

8. Where practicable, all combustibles will be relocated at least 35 feet from the work site. Where relocation is impracticable, combustibles will be protected with flameproofed covers or otherwise shielded with metal or asbestos guards or curtains.

9. Ducts and conveyor systems that might carry sparks to distant combustibles will be suitably protected or shut down.

10. Where cutting or welding is done near walls, partitions, ceiling, or roof of combustible construction, fire-resistant shields or guards will be used.

11. If welding is to be done on a metal wall, partition, ceiling, or roof, precautions will be taken to prevent ignition of combustibles on the other side due to conduction or radiation, preferably by relocating combustibles. Where combustibles are not relocated, a fire watch on the opposite side from the work will be provided.

12. Welding will not be attempted on a metal partition, wall, ceiling, or roof having a combustible covering nor on walls or partitions of combustible sandwich-type panel construction. Cutting or welding on pipes or other metal in contact with combustible walls, partitions, ceilings, or roofs will not be undertaken if the work is close enough to cause ignition by conduction.

13. No welding, cutting, or other hotwork will be performed on used drums, barrels, tanks, or other containers until they have been cleaned so thoroughly as to make absolutely certain that there are no flammable materials present or any substances such as greases, tars, acids, or other materials that, when subjected to heat, might produce flammable or toxic vapors. Any pipelines or connections to the drum or vessel will be disconnected or blanked.

14. All hollow spaces, cavities, or containers will be vented to permit the escape of air or gases before preheating, cutting, or welding.

15. When arc welding is to be suspended for any substantial period of time, all electrodes will be removed from the holders and the holders carefully located so that accidental contact cannot occur; the machine will be disconnected from the power source.

16. In order to prevent the possibility of gas escaping through leaks or improperly closed valves when gas welding or cutting, the torch valves will be closed and the gas supply to the torch positively shut off at some point outside the confined area whenever the torch is not to be used for a substantial period of time. Where practicable, the torch and hose will also be removed from the confined space.

CHAPTER 9

ELECTRICAL SAFETY-RELATED WORK PRACTICES

BACKGROUND

A common misconception in companies is that electrical safety is and should be the sole concern of electricians. In fact, the vast majority of companies do not employ electricians, except through the periodic services of electrical contractors. The typical exposure to electrical hazard in the workplace involves, rather, the worker who comes into contact with electrical conductors in the progress of work that is not characterized as "electrical work" in the same sense that wiring a building or installing an electrical circuit is "electrical work." In some instances, the worker is (or should be) well aware that a particular job entails electrical hazard—as, for example, in the maintenance of equipment or machinery that contains electrical components; however, many workers can become exposed to electrical hazard without recognizing the danger.

In the United States, safety-related work practices regarding electricity, as promulgated by 29 CFR 1910.331–335, pertain to two categories of workers—those who, by the nature of their work (e.g., maintenance), can expect to work on or near an electrical hazard and all other personnel who may accidentally become exposed to electrical hazard. The regulations assume that the former, known as "qualified persons," have received specific training in electrical safety; the latter, known as "unqualified persons," none. The purpose of the regulations is to establish minimum performance standards for both categories of personnel.

As in the case of other HSE regulations, there is much diversity regarding in-plant responsibility for compliance with these electrical safety regulations. While many companies assign primary responsibility to the maintenance supervisor, this approach should be carefully evaluated because of the typically limited authority of a maintenance supervisor regarding the wide range of personnel who are, under these regulations, unqualified persons. A more effective approach is to assign overall responsibility to the person who has more plantwide authority, such as a safety or regulatory compliance officer or human resource manager.

SCOPE

The development of an effective written electrical safety program (Table 9.1) requires completion of a comprehensive electrical audit of a company, with special emphasis on the following aspects:

1. Structural components and features of the plant that describe the source, distribution and use of electrical energy, such as power sources, transformers, circuits, power panels, distribution lines, and electrically operated equipment and machines;

2. Specific job tasks normally performed by personnel that may result in direct contact with live circuits or stored electrical energy, including actions and activities not usually associated with electrical work (e.g., extending a hand into a blind area of a piece of equipment that may contain a live electrical wire);

3. Potential electrical exposures that might occur as a result of non-routine conditions, such as emergency situations (e.g., fire, flood), operational shut-down, and new construction;

4. Potential electrical exposures related to the on-site activity of contractor personnel, including exposures of contractor personnel as well as company employees.

Even where relevant regulations provide for specific exemptions (e.g., in the United States, exemptions for certain types of installations, such as telecommunication installations that are subject to other regulations), the safety officer is well advised to conduct an exhaustive audit of all electrical-related aspects of company facilities and operations. Once all structurally, operationally, and behaviorally related hazards are known, regulatory options can then be exercised in light of not only the potential for regulatory liability but also other types of legal liability (e.g., common law) as well as ethical and moral standards.

TRAINING

While the importance of performance-based training in any aspect of workplace health and safety cannot be overstressed, it is appropriate to note

TABLE 9.1   Major Topics to Be Included in a Written Electrical Safety Program

Electrical Safety Program
Table of Contents

1.   **Introduction**

2.   **Qualified and Unqualified Personnel: Criteria**

3.   **Training**
   - Personnel Requirements
   - Responsibilities

4.   **General Work Practices**
   - All Personnel
   - Qualified Personnel
   - Unqualified Personnel

5.   **Selection and Use of Work**
         Practices (29 CFR 1910.333)
   - Deenergized Parts
   - Energized Parts
   - Overhead Lines
   - Vehicular and Mechanical Equipment
   - Illumination
   - Confined or Enclosed Work Spaces
   - Conductive Materials and Equipment
   - Electrical Interlocks

6.   **Use of Equipment (29 CFR 1910.334)**
   - Portable Electric Equipment
   - Electric Power and Lighting Circuits
   - Test Instruments and Equipment
   - Flammable or Ignitable Materials

7.   **Safeguards for Personal**
         Protection (29 CFR 1910.335)
   - Personal Protective Equipment
   - Protective Tools
   - Alerting Techniques

Appendix 1: List of Qualified Employees
Appendix 2: List of Unqualified Employees

that, in respect to electrical safety, any failure in training will most likely become manifest in dramatic fashion. While inappropriate workplace behavior may result in a worker's receiving simply an electrical shock with little if any aftereffect, such a mild rebuke to either ignorance or lack of concentration or poor judgment is hardly to be considered the norm. Death by electrocution is by far the most frequent workplace consequence of poor training in electrical safety.

Because all personnel should fully understand and be proficient in the prudent electrical safety aspects of all their job tasks, the safety officer must ensure that training in electrical safety is job-specific. This is most often accomplished by gearing training programs to the categories of personnel included in pertinent regulations (i.e., qualified and unqualified personnel), but this approach is often insufficient because such categories are only broadly generic to the degree of electrical risk and not specific to actual and diverse job-related tasks.

For example, under the electrical safety regulations, qualified personnel must receive training in the following:

- skills and techniques necessary to distinguish exposed electrically live parts from other parts of electrical equipment,
- skills and techniques necessary to determine the nominal voltage of exposed electrically live parts, and
- requirements dictated by prudent practice regarding the spatial separation between sources of various voltages and electrically conductive tools (e.g., between a transmission line carrying 750 V and a stepladder).

However, qualified persons who perform maintenance on a company's laboratory instruments and those who perform maintenance on the same company's production equipment have greatly different needs regarding precisely what they have to know, what tools they have to use, and what precautions they have to take.

Similarly, the category "unqualified persons" under these regulations is inclusive of such diverse personnel as a production line worker, a painter, a secretary, and a computer programmer. While there are certainly common informational needs about electrical safety among these workers, more importantly there are also different needs that derive from their specific work environment and their work-related tasks.

In addition to ensuring that training be oriented to the specific job performed by both qualified and unqualified personnel, the safety officer should also carefully consider the potential legal implications that may pertain to training qualified personnel. After all, by definition, qualified personnel are expected to perform company-required work in potentially electrically hazardous situations. Because of the elevated safety risk associated with qualified personnel, it is strongly recommended that the safety officer consider requiring that all training of qualified personnel be conducted by a licensed professional electrician.

Many companies require that the licensed electrician who conducts the training certify qualified personnel by means of their performance on a written examination devised and administered by that licensed electrician. While such "certification" may or may not have relevance in any legal proceeding, it does establish a rational basis for documenting a company's good faith effort to provide high-risk employees with a commensurate level of training.

Finally, the safety officer is best advised that any equipment used in training (e.g., voltage or "tickle" meters; nonconductive clothing, tools, or devices) is precisely the equipment used on-site. In many instances, this practical requirement means that the company must purchase new items as recommended by an instructor who can demonstrate (in writing) that such items are commonly deemed professionally appropriate.

GENERAL WORK PRACTICES

In addition to those work practices specific to individual jobs are those prudent work practices that generally apply to broad categories of workers that might come into contact with electrical hazards.

All Personnel

All personnel, regardless of job function or of status as qualified or unqualified personnel should be subject to the following constraints:

1. No employee may reach blindly into any work area, machine, or equipment that may contain an exposed (i.e., unguarded) electrical hazard;

2. All work potentially involving electrical hazard must be performed in precise conformity with the requirements of the company's energy control (lockout–tagout; Chapter 7) and confined space and hotwork permit (Chapter 8) programs;

3. No person may perform any housekeeping duties where there is electrical hazard unless specifically authorized to do so; in the absence of such authorization, employees must maintain a 10-foot distance from an exposed electrical hazard; and

4. Electrically conductive cleaning materials (e.g., steel wool, conductive liquids) may not be used in proximity to an electrical hazard unless documented procedures are followed that will prevent electrical contact;

where safe work procedures are not in place or commonly used, the employee must coordinate with the corporate safety officer for direction.

Qualified Personnel

In addition to all other requirements imposed by a consideration of the electrical hazards associated with their jobs, the following requirements apply to all qualified personnel:

1. No qualified person may perform any testing of electrical circuits unless specifically authorized and trained to do so.
2. No employee may perform any task in the immediate vicinity (within 10 feet) of an exposed electrical hazard where lack of illumination or an obstruction precludes observation of the work to be performed.
3. No employee may enter any space containing an exposed electrical hazard unless that space is properly illuminated.
4. When working in an enclosed or confined space that contains an exposed electrical hazard, protective shields, barriers, or insulation must be used to prevent inadvertent contact with that hazard. Doors, hinged panels, and the like must be secured to prevent their swinging into the employee and causing inadvertent contact with energized parts.
5. Conductive materials and equipment that are in contact with any part of an employee's body will be handled in such a manner to prevent them from contacting exposed energized conductors or circuits.
6. Portable ladders must be nonconductive if they are used where the employee or the ladder could contact an exposed electrical hazard.
7. Conductive clothing or articles of jewelry may not be worn by employees if they might contact an exposed electrical hazard.

Unqualified Personnel

Under no circumstances will any unqualified person:

1. Work on or near (i.e., within 10 feet of) an exposed electrical hazard;
2. Work on tagged out energized parts of circuits;
3. Open electrical cabinets, switch boxes, or similar devices;
4. Replace, repair, or adjust electrical interlocks, selector switches, control circuits, or power on/off switches;
5. Repair, modify, or install any equipment involving an electrical hazard.

SPECIFIC WORK PRACTICES

It is expected that a written electrical safety program will include specific work practices, procedures, and policies to be employed throughout the facility to prevent electrical shock or other injuries resulting from either direct or indirect electrical contact when work is performed near or on equipment or circuits that may be energized. Examples of such practices, procedures, and policies, which are based on regulatory requirements (29 CFR 1910.331–335), include the following:

Deenergized Parts

Electrically live parts of equipment or machinery to which an employee may be exposed must be deenergized before the employee works on or near them—unless deenergizing introduces additional or increased hazards (e.g., deactivation of alarm system, shut-off of illumination) or is not feasible because of equipment design or operational limits (e.g., testing of electrical circuits that can only be performed with the circuit energized). Live parts that operate at less than 50 V to ground will not be deenergized if there is no increased exposure to electrical burns or to explosion.

Prior to performing any work that can expose personnel to electrical hazard, the person performing that work must ensure compliance with all corporate requirements of energy control (lockout–tagout; Chapter 7) and confined space entry and hotwork (Chapter 8).

Energized Parts

If exposed live parts are not deenergized (according to above criteria), other safety-related work practices must be used to protect employees who may be exposed to the electrical hazards involved. Such work practices will protect employees against contact with energized circuit parts directly with any part of their body or indirectly through some other conductive objective. The work practices used must be suitable for the work performance conditions and for the voltage level of the exposed electrical conductors or circuit parts.

Only "qualified persons" may work on electrical circuit parts or equipment that have not been deenergized in accordance with the corporate energy control program. Such persons must be capable of working safely on energized circuits and will be familiar with the proper use of special precautionary techniques, personal protective equipment, insulating and shielding materials, and insulated tools.

Overhead Lines

If work is to be performed near overhead lines, the lines must be deenergized and grounded, or other protective measures will be provided before work is started. If the lines are to be deenergized, appropriate arrangements to do so must be made with the persons or organization that operates or controls the electrical circuits involved. If protective measures such as guarding, isolating, or insulating are provided, these precautions must prevent employees from contacting electrical lines either directly (i.e., with the body) or indirectly (through other conductors).

When an unqualified person is working in an elevated position near overhead lines, the location will be such that the person and the longest conductive object he or she may contact cannot come closer to any unguarded, energized overhead line than the following distances:

- for voltages to ground $\leq$ 50 kV, 10 feet
- for voltages to ground $>$ 50 kV, 10 feet plus 4 inches for every 10 kV over 50 kV

Under no circumstances will an unqualified person bring any conductive object closer to unguarded, energized overhead lines than the above distances.

When a qualified person is working in the vicinity of overhead lines, whether in an elevated position or on the ground, that person may not approach or take any conductive object without an approved handle closer to exposed energized parts than the following distances:

- $\leq$ 300 V, avoid contact
- $>$ 300 V and $\leq$ 750 V, 1 foot
- $>$ 750 V and $\leq$ 2 kV, 1.5 feet
- $>$ 2 kV and $\leq$ 15 kV, 2 feet
- $>$ 15 kV and $\leq$ 37 kV, 3 feet
- $>$ 37 kV and $\leq$ 87.5 kV, 3.5 feet
- $\geq$ 87.5 kV and $\leq$ 121 kV, 4 feet
- $>$ 121 kV and $\leq$ 140 kV, 4.5 feet

However, the above spatial restrictions do not apply if (a) the person is insulated from the energized part, or (b) the energized part is insulated both from all other conductive objects at a different potential and from the person, or (c) the person is insulated from all conductive objects at a potential different from that of the energized part.

Vehicular and Mechanical Equipment

Any vehicle or mechanical equipment capable of having parts of its structure elevated near energized overhead lines will be operated so that a clearance of 10 feet is maintained. If the voltage is higher than 50 kV, the clearance must be increased 4 inches for every 10 kV over 50 kV. However, under any of the following conditions, the clearance may be reduced:

1. If the vehicle is in transit with its structure lowered, the clearance may be reduced to 4 feet. If the voltage is higher than 50 kV, the clearance will be increased 4 inches for every 10 kV over 50 kV.
2. If insulating barriers are installed to prevent contact with the lines, and if the barriers are rated for the voltage of the line being guarded and are not a part of (or an attachment to) the vehicle or its raised structure, the clearance may be reduced to a distance within the designed working dimensions of the insulating barrier.
3. If the equipment is an aerial lift insulated for the voltage involved, and if the work is performed by a qualified person, the clearance (between the uninsulated portion of the aerial lift and the power line) may be reduced to the distances tabulated above.

No employee standing on the ground may be in direct contact with the vehicle or mechanical equipment or any of its attachments unless:

1. The employee is using protective equipment rated for the voltage, or
2. The equipment is located so that no uninsulated part of its structure can come closer to the line than

- if < 50 kV, then 10 feet
- if > 50 kV, then 10 feet plus 4 inches for every 10 kV over 50 kV

Conductive Materials and Equipment

Conductive materials and equipment that are in contact with any part of an employee's body will be handled in a manner that will prevent contact with exposed energized conductors or circuits. If an employee must handle long dimensional conductive objects (e.g., ducts and pipes) in any area having exposed live parts, the safety officer will ensure that proper insulation, guarding, and/or handling techniques will be implemented to minimize the hazard.

Portable ladders will have nonconductive siderails if they are used where the employee or the ladder could contact exposed energized parts. Conductive articles of jewelry and clothing (e.g., watch bands, bracelets, rings, key chains, necklaces, metalized gloves or aprons, cloth with conductive thread, or metal headgear) will not be worn if they might contact exposed energized parts.

Interlocks

Only a qualified person may defeat an electrical safety interlock, and then only temporarily during the progress of work. The interlock system must be returned to its operable condition when work is completed.

Electrical Cords

Electric cords (including extension cords) may not be used for raising or lowering equipment. Electrical cords may not be fastened with staples or otherwise hung in such a fashion as could damage the other jacket or insulation.

All electric cords must be visually inspected before use for external defects (such as loose parts, deformed and missing pins, or damage to outer jacket or insulation) and for evidence of possible internal damage (such as pinched or crushed outer jacket). If there is a defect or evidence of damage, the cord must be removed from service, and no employee may use it until repairs and tests have rendered it safe and serviceable.

When an attachment plug is to be connected to a receptacle (including any extension cord), the relationship of the plug and receptacle contacts will first be checked to ensure that they are of proper mating configurations. An extension cord used with grounding-type equipment will contain an equipment grounding conductor.

Attachment plugs and receptacles will not be connected or altered in any manner that would prevent proper continuity of the equipment grounding conductor at the point where plugs are attached to receptacles. Also, these devices will not be altered to allow the grounding pole of a plug to be inserted into slots intended for connection to the current-carrying conductors.

Electric cords to be used in highly conductive work locations (such as those inundated with water) or in job locations where employees are likely to contact conductive liquids must be specifically approved by the safety officer.

Power and Lighting Circuits

Load-rated switches, circuit breakers, or other devices specifically designed as disconnecting devices will be used for the opening, reversing, or closing of circuits under load conditions. Cable connectors not of the load-break type, fuses, terminal lugs, and cable splice connections may not be used for such purposes, except in an emergency.

After a circuit is deenergized by a circuit protective device, the circuit may not be manually reenergized until it has been determined that the equipment and circuit can be safely energized. The repetitive manual reclosing of circuit breakers or reenergizing circuits through replaced fuses is strictly prohibited. When it can be determined from the design of the circuit and the overcurrent devices involved that the automatic operation of a device was caused by an overload rather than a fault condition, no examination of the circuit or connected equipment is needed before the circuit is reenergized.

Test Instruments and Equipment

Only qualified persons may perform testing work on electric circuits or equipment. Test instruments and equipment and all associated test leads, cables, power cords, probes, and connectors will be visually inspected for external defects and damage before use. If there is a defect or evidence of damage that may expose an employee to injury, the defective item will be removed from service.

Test instruments and equipment and their accessories will be rated for the circuits and equipment to which they will be connected and will be designed for the environment in which they will be used.

Flammable or Ignitable Materials

Electrical equipment capable of igniting flammable or other ignitable materials will not be used in the vicinity of those materials unless specific measures (e.g., ventilation) are taken to prevent the development of hazardous conditions. All electrical installation requirements for locations where flammable materials are present must be approved by the safety officer after due consultation of pertinent regulations and liaison with local fire authorities.

Personal Protective Equipment

Each employee who works in an area that contains an electrical hazard must be provided protective equipment that is appropriate to the specific parts of the body to be protected and for the work to be performed. Employees must be trained not only in the proper use of protective equipment, but also in the care and maintenance of that equipment, including any prefitting, testing, or inspection that may be required. The safety officer will implement appropriate means for documenting all activities related to prefitting, testing, inspection, and maintenance of protective equipment.

If the electrical insulating capacity of protective equipment may be subject to damage during use, the insulating material will be protected. Employees will wear nonconductive head protection wherever there is a danger of head injury from electrical shock or burns due to contact with exposed energized parts. Employees will wear protective equipment for the eyes or face wherever there is danger of injury to the eyes or face from electrical arcs or flashes or from flying objects resulting from electrical explosion.

General Protective Equipment

When working near exposed electrical hazard, each employee will use insulated tools or handling equipment. Fuse handling equipment, insulated for the circuit voltage, will be used to remove or install fuses when the fuse terminals are energized. Ropes and handlines used near exposed electrical hazards will be nonconductive. Protective shields, protective barriers, or insulating materials will be used to protect each employee from shock, burns, or other electrically related injuries while working near any exposed electrical hazard that might be accidentally contacted or where dangerous electrical heating or arcing might occur. When normally enclosed live parts are exposed for servicing or repair, they will be guarded to protect unqualified persons from contact.

Alerting Techniques

The following alerting techniques will be used to warn and protect employees from hazards that could cause injury due to electrical shock, burns, or failure of electrical equipment parts:

1. Safety signs, safety symbols, or accident prevention tags will be used where necessary throughout the plant to warn employees about electrical hazards. All power panels, fuse boxes, and circuit breakers will be signed to warn employees; these signs will specify voltage and also indicate that access is limited only to authorized personnel.

2. Barricades will be used in conjunction with safety signs where it is necessary to prevent or limit employee access to work areas exposing employees to uninsulated energized conductors. Conductive barricades may not be used where they might cause an electrical contact hazard.

CHAPTER 10

RESPIRATORY PROTECTION

BACKGROUND

As with any type of personal protective equipment, respirators should be considered only when the safety of a workplace atmosphere cannot be maintained by means of other controls (e.g., engineering controls, adjusting work schedules, isolation) or whenever an emergency or interruption in normal atmospheric protection (e.g., servicing of ventilation motors) results in respiratory hazard.

In the United States, the use of workplace respirators is governed by 29 CFR 1910.134, which requires the development of a written respiratory protection program. While responsibilities regarding the respiratory protection program are often shared by a variety of personnel, including production and operations managers and those employees designated to wear respirators, overall responsibility for the development, implementation, and oversight of relevant procedures is typically given to a corporate safety officer.

For the purpose of designing a respiratory protection program, it is essential that the safety officer understand that a respirator is any device that treats or provides air to be inhaled by its wearer, including as simple a device as a paper dust mask that is commonly available for purchase at retail stores. In general, respirators may be described as being "air-purifying" or "air-supplying"—the former to remove atmospheric contaminants from an atmosphere that otherwise contains sufficient oxygen, the latter to provide a safe source of oxygen. Selecting between these two categories of respirators and from among the many types of each depends not on any so-called "common sense" assessment of relative complexity or simplicity, but on a precise understanding of (a) the nature of the respiratory hazard associated with a particular job and (b) the capabilities, limitations, and even risks of appropriate respiratory protection.

It is also essential that the safety officer understand that neither the need for nor the use of respiratory protection devices can be left to the personal experience, whims, or preferences of the individual worker. The fact that workers do not immediately exhibit adverse health symptoms due to atmospheric contaminants does not mean that respiratory protection is unnecessary; many of the health effects of respired atmospheric contaminants are, after all, chronic and often require even decades to become manifest. As to common complaints regarding "personal discomfort" in wearing respirators or their being "only for sissies," the basic presumption of any legally responsible and morally defensible health and safety program must be that the level of personal protection is to be determined solely by the job and its associated hazard. Wherever the requisites of health and safety and the preferences of the individual worker are dissonant, it is the health and safety requisites that must prevail.

RESPIRATORY HAZARDS

Common air contaminants include a variety of solid and liquid "particles" that range greatly in size, from relatively large-sized liquid chemical mists (>100 μm) to progressively smaller particles, like dusts (e.g., foundry dust and fly ash [1–1000 μm]), fumes and vapors (e.g., metallurgical fumes and oil smoke [0.001–1.0 μm]), and, finally, gases. The size of an inhaled particle is a key factor in the depth to which that particle can penetrate into the respiratory tract. While the depth of penetration is also influenced greatly by the shape of the particles and whether inhalation is primarily through the nose or the mouth, the majority of larger dusts and mists can become deposited along the nasopharyngeal portion of the respiratory tract (above the larynx and including nasal passages); with progressively smaller particles progressing to the upper esophagus, to the tracheobronchial branches of the respiratory tract and, finally, even to the alveoli of the lung. Particles deposited in nasal passages and within the throat can also ultimately enter the stomach via passage along the esophagus—demonstrating that inhalation, as a route of entry (Chapter 3), can be equivalent to that other route of entry, ingestion.

Given the range of potential deposition of inhaled particles within both the respiratory and gastrointestinal tract, various organs and tissues become exposed to the diverse health hazards associated with those particles, including such relatively mild acute afflictions as nasal irritation (e.g., certain chromium dusts), persistent sneezing (e.g., o-chlorobenzylidene malononitrile), and cough (e.g., chlorine), and life-threatening acute and chronic afflictions as pneumonia (e.g., manganese dusts in lower airways and alveoli), hemorrhage (e.g., boron vapors in alveoli), emphysema (e.g., aluminum abrasives in alveoli), and cancer (e.g., nickel dusts in nasal cavities and the lung).

Upon being inhaled, various gases, vapors, and mists (e.g., halogenated hydrocarbons, methyl ethyl ketone, methyl methacrylate) can pass directly from the alveoli (or from the gastrointestinal tract) into the blood and, depending upon their differential solubilities in different body fluids and tissues (e.g., fat), affect other tissues (e.g., bone), organs (e.g., liver), and systems (e.g., central nervous system). Of course, many air contaminants begin to exert their effect immediately upon entry into the blood by triggering an immunological response. For example, many organic dusts, such as cork, malt, and cheese dust and even organic dusts that collect in air conditioners, as well as inorganic dusts, such as tungsten carbide, platinum salts, toluene 2,4-diisocyanate, and nickel metal dusts, can cause allergenic reactions in hypersensitive persons that can quickly become life threatening. Differential solubilities of air contaminants in body fluids and materials, as well as their potential as immunological antigens, clearly illustrates that many inhaled contaminants are not simply respiratory hazards, but are in fact hazards to the whole body.

JOB HAZARD ANALYSIS FOR RESPIRATORY PROTECTION

While a job hazard analysis (or audit) is a necessary first step toward the development of any health and safety program, it is worthwhile to highlight those elements of job hazard analysis that are particularly relevant to developing a respiratory protection plan.

Sources of Respiration Hazards

Too often the search for potential sources of workplace respiration hazards is confined solely to a survey of those gases, fumes, vapors, dusts, and mists that are generated in production processes. While this is a necessary consideration, it is only one of a number of appropriate considerations. A more exhaustive search would include all of the following potential sources of atmospheric risks in the workplace:

1. Materials produced in unit processes directly related to production, including contaminants created by such activities as

- processing stock materials, as in grinding, cutting, sanding, polishing, mixing, reacting, spraying, heating, and treating raw materials and finished products

- handling raw materials, as in charging and discharging silos, loading stock bins and reactors, and transporting stock via bulk containers, conveyor belts, and chutes

2. Materials contained in the exhausts of vehicles, equipment, and machines, such as

- combustion products in vehicular exhaust
- air exhausts from bag houses, cyclones, and ventilation units

3. Materials entrained in plant atmosphere from nonproduction plant activities or structures, including

- maintenance activities
- housekeeping and grounds management (e.g., painting, application of pesticides, fertilization of lawns, operation of decorative fountains)
- new construction and structural repair or refurbishment
- build-up of dusts in ventilation shafts and ducts

4. Materials entrained in plant atmosphere from other sources, such as

- local vehicular traffic
- atmospheric contamination from other workplaces, including industrial, commercial, and agricultural facilities

5. Deficiency in oxygen due to

- displacement of air by heavier chemical vapors and gases (asphyxiants) in confined spaces, including ditches, subfloor spaces, underground vaults, tanks and reactions vessels, sewers, and silos
- consumption of air due to decomposition of organic materials (mineralization) by bacteria and other microbes, as in enclosed storage facilities for organic materials and sewer conduits

In undertaking such a comprehensive survey, the safety officer is best advised to utilize a committee composed of employees from different departments. Such a committee embodies extensive practical experience with the total physical plant and its environs.

Exposure Analysis

Having identified potential sources of atmospheric risks, the next step is to determine precisely which employees are at risk with respect to each

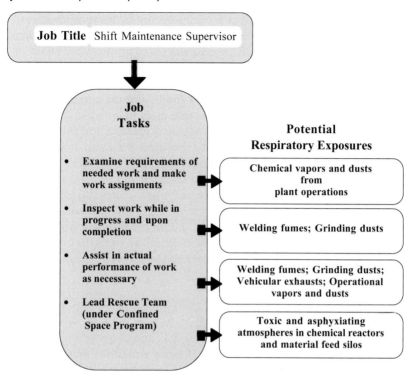

FIGURE 10.1 A job title usually defines a series of specific job tasks, each of which may result in respiratory risk. An effective respiratory protection program must therefore be based on a precise understanding of all the tasks associated with a particular type of job and how each task may contribute to an individual worker's respiratory risk.

source and to what degree such exposures warrant the use of respiratory protection devices.

The objective here is to define actual linkages between persons and atmospheric contaminants that may occur under a range of workday circumstances, including (a) normal or routine operations, (b) nonroutine situations, such as power outages and unit shutdown, and (c) emergency situations, such as fire, flood, or high wind. These linkages are usually not immediately evident in the job titles of personnel; they are manifest, rather, in the nature and location of specific tasks that employees perform under routine, nonroutine, and emergency situations (Figure 10.1).

It is crucial that ambient monitoring with regard to potential sources of atmospheric contaminants not be implemented until individual employees at risk are identified. This approach, which is clearly in opposition to the usual practice of ambient monitoring programs that tend to focus on "places," ensures that the focus of monitoring becomes "persons-in-places." While ambient monitoring is discussed in detail in Chapter 16, it is sufficient to emphasize here that all too often measurements of atmospheric contaminants have little relevance to the quality of air actually inhaled by individual workers because they fail to represent such factors as the relative vapor density of chemicals, the air dynamics of a room, and the actual schedules and work habits of individuals. The basic rule must be to conduct ambient monitoring (a) when the potential for exposure is greatest and (b) precisely where those exposures occur, whether it be throughout a room, in a cabinet, 3 inches from the floor, or next to the ceiling—wherever a worker's nose may become the route-of-entry for a hazardous contaminant.

This "under-the-nose" approach to ambient monitoring, especially if conducted with meticulous concern for the different circumstances of routine, nonroutine, and emergency situations and for the different work schedules and habits of individual workers, should allow the safety officer to establish a "worst case" estimate of worker exposure to atmospheric hazard.

Action Levels

In the broad context of industrial hygiene, an *action level* is usually a numerical limit (but it may also be a qualitative situation) that triggers a protective response. In some few cases, action levels may be established by regulations pertaining to specific chemicals, such as benzene or formaldehyde. In most instances, action levels are established by common practice. For example, in most companies having a comprehensive health and safety program, evacuation from an area containing flammable vapors is required whenever ambient concentrations attain 10% of the lower explosive limit (LEL). The rationale for any action limit is that protection must begin well in advance of an actual life- or health-threatening situation.

In the absence of either an action level or even so much as a standard or guideline established by legal authority (which are by far the most common situations), the safety officer must nonetheless establish a criterion for deciding whether or not the measured quality of an atmosphere requires the use of respiratory protection. Sometimes, given the dearth of action levels and standards as compared with the seemingly limitless number of health and safety hazards, the safety officer opts to require respiratory protection regardless of ambient concentrations. This practice, however, must be strongly discouraged because the use of any protective clothing or devices always carries with it its own risk. The objective should be to balance the risks that derive from the lack of specific protection with the risks that derive from wearing protective equipment, such as those attendant to a false sense of security and equipment failure.

Lacking legally promulgated action levels or other professional guidance, the safety officer is better advised to establish an action level that is both practicable and clearly reflective of the fact that, assuming that all practicable controls (e.g., engineering controls, scheduling, isolation, rotation of personnel) have been adequately considered and implemented, a company-required protective respiratory device becomes the last remaining protection between the worker and possibly lethal injury.

While the 10% rule in common industrial use regarding explosive vapors is a stringent rule, it is not at all unreasonable to consider extrapolating it to other circumstances. In a situation involving an atmospheric contaminant for which there is a standard (TLV) of, for example, 4.0 mg/m^3, this rule would establish a worst case exposure of 0.4 mg/m^3 as being the trigger for requiring respiratory protection.

In the absence of a relevant legal standard, and as long as such an action level does not conflict with commonly accepted prudent professional practice regarding the contaminant of concern, the 10% criterion is arguably responsive to both the goal of workplace health and safety and the need for a practicable means for achieving that goal. However, it must be reiterated that under no circumstance, including the lack of a legal standard or action level, may any consideration of practicability, however measured by cost, ready availability, or personal comfort or any other factor, result in a degree of respiratory protection that is less than that required by the state-of-art professional practice of industrial hygiene. The measure of "correctness" is ultimately what "the best among us" are doing. Sometimes, this state-of-art emulation requires not only the use of an admittedly stringent action level, but also the adoption of other practices that elevate safety margins. For example, some companies (including some manufacturers of respiratory protection devices) require that, prior to applying action level criteria to worst-case measurements of the ambient concentration of an atmospheric contaminant, the worst-case measurements be first multiplied by a safety factor of two or more.

TYPES OF RESPIRATORS

Any reputable manufacturer or supplier of respirators today offers potential clients detailed documentation regarding the broad range of available respirators and the specific uses and limits of each type. Under no circumstance should the safety officer purchase any respirator without carefully examining this documentation or without consulting with manufacturers' or suppliers' technical staffs.

The basic types of respiratory protection devices (Figure 10.2) may be briefly described as follows.

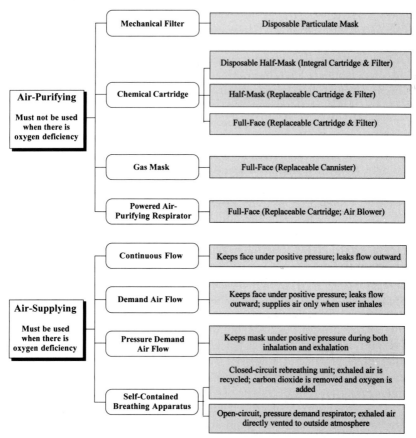

FIGURE 10.2 Typology of respirators (adapted from information provided by Jean Letendre). Each respirator has specific limitations and requirements that must be assessed in light of job-specific circumstances.

Air-Purifying Respirators

These respirators use filter and/or sorbent materials to remove contaminants from inhaled air. These respirators must not be used in atmospheres that may have either a deficiency (<19.5%) or an excess (>22.5%) of oxygen.

1. Mechanical filter respirator: Removes particles from the air; consists of a simple mesh material that fits over the nose and mouth and is tied with straps or strings behind the neck; a comfortable, low-profile, lightweight respirator (often called simply a "paper" or "dust mask") for limited

use; low-cost protection against dust, mist, and fumes, but not effective for gases, vapors, or nonabsorbed contaminants; no cleaning, disinfection, or spare parts required; the usual limit for use is set at 10 times the permissible exposure limit (PEL).

2. Chemical cartridge respirator: Either a disposable half-face respirator in which the cartridge is integral to the facepiece or a nondisposable half- or full-face respirator with one or two screw-on chemical cartridges that are specific for particular contaminants; use limited by ambient concentration of contaminants; expended cartridges may be replaced; easy to use; needs little cleaning and few if any spare parts; protection against gas, vapor, dust, and mists; limit is usually set at 10 times the PEL (but may be different) and is indicated on the cartridge.

3. Gas mask: A full-face mask to which is attached a relatively long-lived canister containing sorbent materials that can remove toxic gases and particles; expended canisters may be replaced; offers a greater capacity for removing high ambient concentrations of contaminants than cartridge respirators; limits for ambient concentrations are specified on the canister.

4. Powered air-purifying respirator: A helmeted, hooded, or full-face mask containing one or more cartridges through which air is forced by an air blower; less exhausting for user than chemical cartridge or gas mask respirators; face- or belt-mounted blower that is battery powered; limits are usually set at 100 times the PEL (or as specified on the cartridge).

Air-Supplying Respirators

These respirators consist of a helmet, hood, full- or half-face mask that is provided air through a compressor or compressed air cylinder. They are used in atmosphere that may have a deficiency or an excess of oxygen, or the concentration of contaminant vapors, gases, or particles may be immediately dangerous to life or beyond the capacity of an air-purifying cartridge or canister.

1. Continuous flow respirator: The facepiece is kept at positive pressure; air flow is outward from the mask, preventing contaminants from entering the facepiece; supplies clean, breathable air from a source independent of the contaminated air; the flow of air remains constant.

2. Demand air flow respirator: Supplies air only when the user inhales; exhalations are ejected directly to the atmosphere; flow of air is regulated by pressure valve.

3. Pressure demand air flow respirator: Supplies air when the user inhales or exhales; exhalations are ejected directly to the atmosphere; flow of air is regulated by pressure valve.

4. Self-contained breathing apparatus (SCBA): Provides an independent air supply that is not mixed with the outside atmosphere and which may be either recycled or exhaled directly into the outside atmosphere; offers greatest respiratory protection available.

GENERAL PROCEDURES

The written respiratory protection program must include specific procedures that govern the use of respirators throughout the workplace. Many of these procedures assign various responsibilities which, of course, may vary from company to company, to specific personnel. The following examples illustrate the range of issues that must be addressed and adapted to the specific managerial practices of any company:

1. Respirators will be selected on the basis of the specific hazards to which individual employees may be exposed in normal, nonroutine, and emergency situations. While the selection of respirators is finally the responsibility of the safety officer, the safety officer will coordinate with all department managers having employees identified as in need of respiratory protection.

2. Only personnel authorized by the safety officer will utilize respirators. Authorization consists of (a) selection by the safety officer on the basis of potential exposure to dangerous atmospheres, (b) appropriate training of selected personnel in the proper use, maintenance, and limitations of the specific respirator specified for their use, and (c) completion of medical evaluation and fit testing requirements.

3. All authorized personnel identified in this program will be trained in the proper fitting of respirators and taught how to conduct fit testing. All managers of departments in which personnel use any type of respirator will be fully trained in all aspects regarding the proper use, maintenance, and fitting of respirators.

4. The safety officer will ensure that whenever possible, training of personnel and managers will be conducted by the company's vendors of respiratory protection devices and will maintain all training records, including the date of training, the names of persons attending the training, the specific subject matter addressed, and the name and affiliation of the trainer.

5. Wherever possible, respirators will be assigned to individual workers for their exclusive use; in such cases, the employee's name will be clearly marked on the respirator.

6. All respirators must be cleaned and disinfected after each use and will be stored in a convenient, clean, sanitary, and clearly identified location.

Written instructions for the proper cleaning, disinfection, storage, and maintenance of respirators will be included in standard operating procedures posted at each location.

7. Respirators will be inspected during cleaning or at least monthly. Worn or deteriorated parts will be replaced. Inspection will include a check of the tightness of connections and the condition of the facepiece, headbands, valves, connecting tubes, and canisters. Rubber or elastomer parts will be inspected for pliability and signs of deterioration. Inspection records will be maintained by departmental supervisors at the respirator storage location.

8. Respirators must be stored to protect against dust, sunlight, heat, extreme cold, excessive moisture, or damaging chemicals. Respirators placed at stations and work areas for emergency use will be immediately accessible at all times and should be stored in dedicated and clearly signed compartments. Routinely used respirators, such as dust masks, may be placed in plastic bags for storage. Respirators should not be stored in such places as lockers or tool boxes unless they are in carrying cases or cartons.

9. Respirators should be packed or stored so that the facepiece and exhalation valve will rest in a normal position and function will not be impaired by the elastomer setting in an abnormal position.

10. All personnel who issue or use canister-type respirators will ensure that canisters purchased or used by them are properly labeled and colored (in accordance with 29 CFR 1910.134, Table I-1) before they are placed in service and that labels and colors are properly maintained at all times thereafter.

11. The safety officer will ensure that work areas and operations requiring the use of respirators are monitored at least twice a year to ensure proper respiratory protection. The safety officer will maintain written records that document the date of monitoring, chemical monitored, measurement devices, concentrations, conversion factors, mathematical transformations of data, as well as any actions undertaken as a result of the monitoring effort.

12. In the case of SCBA, air may be supplied to respirators from cylinders or air compressors only if in compliance with 29 CFR 1910.134(d).

13. In areas where the wearer of a respiratory protection device could, upon failure of that device, be overcome by a toxic or oxygen deficiency or superabundance, at least one additional person will be present. Communications will be maintained between both or all individuals present. Planning will be such that one individual will be unaffected by any likely incident and have the proper rescue equipment to effect rescue.

14. Personnel using air line respirators in atmospheres immediately hazardous to life or health will be equipped with safety harnesses and safety lines for lifting or removing persons from hazardous atmospheres.

15. Under no circumstances will an authorized employee wear eye contact lenses in any atmosphere that may be chemically contaminated.

EVALUATION OF AUTHORIZED PERSONNEL

All personnel to be authorized for the use of respirators must first be medically evaluated by a licensed physician to determine their fitness to use the selected respirator. The physician has sole responsibility for determining which health and physical conditions are pertinent for this examination.

The medical examination should be conducted at least annually for all authorized personnel. Under no circumstances may any person undertake to wear a respirator of any type without a written determination by the attending physician that the person is medically fit to wear the specific respirator under the conditions of its intended use.

Finally, no person can be authorized to work with a respirator who has not successfully met the fit testing requirements for that respirator. This requirement is absolute and cannot be set aside by any consideration of a personal attribute (e.g., facial contour and structure, facial hair) that precludes successful fit testing.

CHECKLIST FOR AUTHORIZED PERSONNEL

In addition to the specific assignments of responsibility to the safety officer and other managerial personnel, the written respiratory protection program should clearly identify the responsibilities of personnel who actually wear the respiratory protection devices. These responsibilities are often most usefully reiterated by a check list provided to authorized personnel that contains such entries as the following:

- Inspect for any structural damage both before and after use. After use, clean and disinfect the respirator according to the written SOP.
- In case of structural damage, discard the item and replace with a new unit. Do not make repairs.
- Do not alter the respirator in any way.
- To ensure proper protection, perform the fit test each time you use the respirator.
- Use the respirator only for the use specified in the written SOP. Be sure that you understand the limitations of the respirator you are using.
- Store the respirator only as directed in the written SOP.

- Report to your department manager (or the safety officer) in the event of any problems with your health or with your respirator.

OTHER DOCUMENTATION

In addition to the documentation maintained regarding job and exposure analyses, medical evaluation of authorized personnel, fit testing and equipment inspection, and ambient air monitoring, a well developed written respiratory protection program will include summaries of key information and SOPs.

For example, it is most useful to maintain an up-to-date table that correlates (a) company departments (e.g., boiler house, analytical laboratory), (b) operations within departments (e.g., pipe fitting and welding, heavy metal analysis), (c) required types of respirators (e.g., toxic mechanical filter), and (d) the names of personnel authorized to use those respirators. Such a tabulation can serve as a basic tool for monitoring in-house compliance with basic requirements of the overall program and also as a guide for reviewing the adequacy of the previously performed jobs analysis.

Also vital, of course, are written SOPs that serve as the key management tools for implementing the program. Usually written in a standard format, these SOPs must be specific to clearly identified job tasks or operations. Examples of the types of information to be included in such SOPs include:

- description of operation
- respirator type required for operation (including make and model number)
- date respirator type was formally designated as a requirement
- name of person authorizing respirator type
- procedures for assembling respirator
- procedures regarding pre-use inspection of respirator
- requirements for respirator maintenance, cleaning, inspection, and storage
- limitations and cautions relevant to use of respiration
- step-by-step procedure for using and fit testing respirator

Finally, the written program must contain a list of the names of authorized personnel. This list, maintained up-to-date, is the basic means for ensuring compliance with the medical evaluation and training requirements regarding authorized personnel and also for conducting on-site program compliance audits.

CHAPTER 11

HEARING CONSERVATION

BACKGROUND

The basic objective of a hearing conservation program is to prevent occupationally induced hearing loss. While a diversity of health effects of noise have been suggested and studied, including effects on mental performance and psychological or physiological well being, hearing loss, which is most often associated with sound-induced physical, physiochemical, or metabolic injury of key cellular components of the inner ear, remains the focus of regulatory standards and protective measures. This is not to argue that other effects such as noise-induced fatigue and dizziness or disorientation (i.e., vertigo) are not real or that they are insignificant aspects of human health, but only that such effects are subsumed under a standard that is essentially oriented toward hearing loss.

The basic rule of thumb is that the louder the noise and the longer a person's exposure to that noise, the greater the potential for hearing loss. The loudness of noise (i.e., intensity, power, amplitude) is measured in terms of decibels (dB), which is a logarithmic unit, with 80 dB commonly accepted as the level of noise that a person can tolerate for 8 hr per day without significant risk of hearing loss.

Amplitude is only one attribute of sound energy that has implication for human health; another attribute of sound that must be considered is the pitch (i.e., frequency) of sound, which is measured in hertz units (Hz), with 1 Hz = 1 cycle per second (cps). The range of human hearing, which is dependent upon frequency, ranges from 2 to 20,000 Hz. Sound meters typically used in the industrial setting measure amplitude at various frequencies or ranges (bands) of frequencies (i.e., at different octaves). Depending upon an instrument's weighting of the loudness of noise at different frequencies, loudness may be expressed simply as dB units (where the power of sounds having different frequencies are equally weighted), or in slightly different units, such as dBA, dBB, and dBC, with the second capitalized letter denoting different schemes of weighting the amplitudes of the different frequencies.

Permissible noise exposures promulgated in the United States by OSHA (29 CFR 1910.95), are based on dBA values, where the "A" indicates that the sound meter is much more sensitive to noise above 1000 Hz, frequencies much more likely to damage the inner ear. The regulated limits clearly reflect concern for the increasing risk of hearing impairment with both increasing duration of exposure and increasing decibel level, ranging from a permissible exposure of 8 hr to 90 dBA to 15 min or less to 115 dBA. When daily noise exposure is composed of two or more periods of noise exposure at different levels, the combined effect must be considered on the basis of a weighted average algorithm.

As with many other aspects of workplace health and safety, including chemical and electrical risk, the workplace is not unique as a source of potentially injurious sound. The sound level of a club band can exceed that of many industrial machines; the sound level of various industrial drills and presses is on the order of the sound level of a power mower. However, the critical difference between noise in the industrial setting as opposed to that experienced in home, community, and recreational settings is most often the significantly longer duration of workplace exposure to potentially injurious levels.

NOISE REDUCTION STRATEGIES

A wide variety of different strategies for reducing the level of noise or the duration of a worker's exposure to injurious levels is available, including (in order of priority) engineering control strategies, managerial practices, and the use of personal protective equipment.

Engineering control, beginning at the source of potentially harmful noise and progressing to the control of the transmission of noise within the workplace, includes such measures as the following:

- Preference given to the selection and purchase of that machinery which, in comparison with machinery otherwise having equal functional value, is structurally equipped or otherwise designed to minimize the generation of noise or dampen its transmission
- On-site reengineering of machine and equipment to minimize noise generation or transmission by employing vibration absorbent materials (footing cushions and springs), noise damping agents (e.g., paints and coatings, panel pads), and muffling devices (e.g., exhaust and intake mufflers)
- Use of physical isolation and structural barriers to restrict noise to specific locations and reduce transmitted noise to workers,

including total and partial enclosures of machines and equipment and the installation of sound barriers and baffles

Managerial practices, which should be considered only after all appropriate engineering control strategies have been implemented, involve practices governing the workplace behavior of personnel, including:

- Rotating personnel or altering personal work schedules to limit the duration of exposure of individual workers to injurious noise
- Altering the staging (i.e., timing or scheduling) of workplace processes that contribute to the cumulative noise level in the workplace
- Controlling access to portions of the workplace, including access by visitors as well as employees and contractors

Personal protective equipment should be considered only after all engineering and managerial practices have been exhausted and only in conformance with the requirements of a written hearing conservation program (HCP).

Usually the responsibility of a corporate safety officer, but also demanding close coordination with plant managers and production personnel, a comprehensive HCP includes policies and procedures regarding (a) ambient noise monitoring, (b) employee rights, (c) audiometric testing, (d) hearing protectors and noise attenuation, (e) employee training, and (f) record keeping.

AMBIENT NOISE MONITORING

Regulations typically describe the trigger for implementing an ambient noise monitoring program as "information indicating" that any employee's exposure may equal or exceed an 8-hr time-weighted average of 85 dB. Unfortunately, many plant managers and even safety officers fail to give proper attention to two key aspects of this description:

First, "any information" includes actual data on noise levels, as well as concerns or complaints of workers. It also includes (and this must be stressed) information generally applicable to comparable workplaces—the so-called "state-of-art" criterion. Too often, the safety officer consciously or subconsciously injects a personal opinion regarding the significance of workplace noise into the determination of the need for a monitoring program. Under no circumstance may a subjective opinion be used to decide that ambient monitoring is not required.

Second, the phrase "any employee" cannot be overemphasized. The objective of a hearing conservation program is to eliminate the threat of workplace-induced injury, not to that nameless collectivity known as "work-

TABLE 11.1   Example of Data Format Used in a Study of Industrial Sound Levels

Global Enterprises, Inc.			Noise Exposure Data Date Collected: July 26, 1996 Collected by: Sound Consultants, Inc.		
Name	**Title**	**Location**	**Task**	**Test Duration**	**Average dBA**
Dorothy Winslow	Machine Operator	Tool Room	Run metal grinder	6 hr 30 min	82
Augustine Lee	Carpenter	Wire Prep Print Shop	Install new shelving Rebuild spread tables	2 hr 15 min 3 hr	70 75
Hans Kirkoffen	Material Handler	Equipment Prep	Load and unload conveyor	7 hr	78
Mahat Sulaiman	Pressman	Print Shop	Operate printing press	7 hr 30 min	76
Donald Oldman	Painter	Paint Shop	Operate spray booth	6 hr 30 min	70
Annette Bilsoy	Welder	Boiler Room Press Room Plating Area	Cut scrape metal plates Pipefitting Pipefitting	3 hr 30 min 1 hr 2 hr 15 min	84 71 65
Raw data used to calculate means are included in Appendix 3. Cumulative exposures by name of employee over period of testing (July 22-August 2) are included in Appendix 4.					**Page 2 of 30**

ers," but to individual persons. Recognizing that the sound level associated with such home appliances as a food blender, garbage disposal, and even a clothes or dishwasher is on the order of 75–85 dB, the safety officer must understand that no personal opinion or commonsense judgment can substitute for the measurement of the actual noise to which each individual worker is exposed in the performance of each job.

In light of these two considerations, and excepting that workplace throughout which noise hardly exceeds the level of normal human conversation (50–60 dB), the safety officer is strongly advised to initiate a monitoring program and to base all subsequent actions on actual monitoring data.

The monitoring program should be designed and conducted by personnel who are thoroughly knowledgeable regarding both regulatory requirements and the technical and scientific methods and instrumentation associated with the measurement of sound. In the vast majority of companies, the design and implementation of the monitoring program is contracted out to a consultant. Even in cases where a corporate safety officer is a certified industrial hygienist and is otherwise fully qualified to perform the monitoring, it is advisable to utilize expertise that is external to the company, if only to obviate even the appearance of undue company influence on how or where measurements are made or on the interpretation of data.

As shown in Table 11.1, a competent monitoring program will include the following types of information:

- the name of specific personnel performing a monitored task
- the in-plant location where the task is performed
- a description of the task monitored
- the duration of the monitoring conducted for that task
- the monitoring data obtained

It is crucial that monitoring be conducted at times that reflect the range of workplace circumstances, including both normal and nonroutine situations, and that the positioning of monitors be such as to reflect the sound levels actually experienced by individual workers. In order to meet these requirements, the consulting specialist must become thoroughly familiar with workplace conditions and operations, including physical layout, types of machines, equipment and processes, job descriptions, and work schedules, prior to designing the monitoring program.

While the primary objective of the monitoring effort is to identify "which persons performing which tasks" are subjected to noise levels requiring amelioration, any well designed program should also identify which sources of unacceptable sound levels may be appropriately ameliorated by engineering and managerial practices. After engineering or managerial correctives have been implemented, these sources should be monitored again to determine if personal hearing protection devices are nonetheless required.

Several additional aspects of ambient monitoring should be given particular attention by the safety officer:

1. Workplace noise is inclusive of two basic categories of sound: (a) *impulsive sound*, which is sound that varies more than 40 dB per 0.5 sec, and (b) *nonimpulsive sound*, which includes so-called *continuous* and *intermittent* (i.e., varies less than 40 dB per 0.5 sec) sound. The monitoring program must integrate all continuous, intermittent, and impulsive sound levels for 80 to 130 dB.

2. While the standard action level for workplace noise is an 8-hr TWA of 85 dB, a well designed monitoring program may nonetheless describe certain job tasks as possibly requiring (as opposed to definitely requiring) correction. This is most often due to one or more of the following reasons: (a) the calculation of the ambient TWA is subject to significant error because it is based on data that were collected over less than an 8-hr interval, (b) the investigator determines that the error inherent in the sensitivity limits, in combination with the actual monitoring duration, produces a statistical confidence level that does not permit a clear decision whether or not a mean dB value meets the action level criterion, and (c) the investigator determines that, even though within the normal methodological error, a final result is, in fact, "borderline" with respect to the legal action level. In all such circumstances, the safety officer should consider borderline data as, in fact, indicative of the need for corrective action.

3. Additional monitoring is required whenever changes in operations or equipment may affect the levels of workplace noise. The most useful rule of thumb (from the perspective of both legal liability and the protection of human health) is to assume that, in the absence of documented monitoring data to the contrary, any operation resulting in noise greater than that associated with normal human conversation exceeds the action level.

EMPLOYEE RIGHTS

Any employee who is exposed to workplace noise at or above the legal action level of 85 dB must be informed of the actual results of the monitoring program. Such an employee, who is referred to as an "affected employee" in the written HCP, also has the right to observe the actual measurement of ambient noise. The intent of these requirements (29 CFR 1910.95 (e) and (f)) is clearly to inform the employee of precisely the hearing risks associated with workplace tasks and the manner by which those risks are evaluated—an intent that is increasingly explicit in health and safety regulations.

Because employees must have access to the results of monitoring data, it should be assumed that they have the right to question and evaluate not only those data, but also the overall design of the monitoring program. This assumption is consonant with the growing recognition that, in all matters of workplace health and safety, employee access to information is essentially equivalent to employee participation in corporate decision-making having direct relevance to their health and safety. While the degree of that participation is certainly subject to much ongoing discussion, controversy, and even legal litigation, there is little question that, today, the employee is much more a partner, along with management, than simply a passive object in any corporate health and safety program. In this regard, the safety officer is well advised to consider the participation of employees in all stages of the monitoring program, from early discussions with the consulting specialist through the review of preliminary and final findings.

AUDIOMETRIC TESTING

The company must provide audiometric testing to affected employees at no cost to those employees. In the United States, regulations include specific requirements regarding the certification of persons performing the audiometric testing, testing devices and methodology, and types and frequency of audiograms (29 CFR 1910.95(g)). While such requirements may vary from nation to nation, certain aspects of audiometric testing should be emphasized as of universal concern:

1. The *baseline audiogram* is a hearing test conducted on an employee shortly following workplace exposure to noise above the action level. As implied by the term "baseline," the objective of this audiogram is to define the normal hearing capacity of the employee in the absence of any workplace-induced impairment. Subsequent audiograms can thereafter be compared with the baseline audiogram to detect work-related hearing impairment and, therefore, the need for appropriate revisions to company policies and practices regarding hearing protection.

Given the importance of the baseline audiogram, it is imperative that it be completed before workplace noise above the action level results in actual hearing impairment. Also, because noise can cause short- as well as long-term hearing impairment (known, respectively, as *temporary threshold shifts* [TTS] and *permanent threshold shifts* [PTS]), it is necessary that the affected worker avoid or otherwise be protected from workplace noise prior to examination for a baseline audiogram. In the United States, the standard requires that the baseline audiogram of an affected employee be established within 6 months (or, where mobile testing vans are utilized for the purpose, within 1 year) of the employee's first exposure at or above the action level and that the employee not be exposed to workplace noise for at least 14 hr immediately preceding the test.

2. Subsequent audiograms should be obtained for affected employees over short enough time intervals to ensure the early detection of hearing impairment. In the United States, the standard rule is that audiograms for affected employees be obtained at least annually. Longer intervals not only lead to an increased risk of permanent threshold shifts in specific individuals, but also deny any effective quality control over the HCP, with possible serious consequences to the hearing of personnel throughout the plant that can, in turn, result in progressively expanding risks not only in employee health and safety but also in corporate litigation.

3. In comparing baseline and subsequent (at least annual) audiograms, the focus is on detecting an impairment of hearing. The action level for such a determination is what is called a *standard threshold shift* which, in the United States, is a change in hearing (relative to the baseline audiogram) of an average of 10 dB or more at 2000, 3000, and 4000 Hz in either ear. American OSHA regulations also provide for (but do not mandate) the standardized adjustment of annual audiograms for the aging process in making the determination of a standard threshold shift.

The safety officer is advised that the decision as to whether or not to adjust annual audiograms for age should not be left to medical judgment alone because this decision has broad implications that go well beyond the professional purview of any attending physician, including:

A. Correcting an annual audiogram for aging is basically equivalent to lessening any observed difference between baseline and annual audiograms, and this, in turn, results in the removal of a possibly desirable safety margin. Of course, by not correcting for age, the safety officer may cause an age-related hearing impairment to be falsely attributed to workplace exposure.

B. The use of any regulatory rule, especially a nonmandated technique (which the American procedure for performing age-adjustments of audiometric data is) does not provide absolute legal protection in a legal tort involving the injury of an employee that may or may not be work related. Any practical corporate gain to be achieved by taking such an option is therefore highly questionable, especially in light of negative public relations likely to be realized for appearing to "use age as an excuse for corporate irresponsibility."

C. Even where there may be good reason to exercise this option, serious consideration should be given to the relevance of the data base used to perform the age adjustment. For example, are the data (even if provided by regulatory authority) biased to particular national, cultural, or other social (including gender) groups? Is the data base current? What is the extent of professional consensus regarding both the utility and the limitations of the data base?

4. Where the comparison of an employee's baseline and annual audiogram reveals a standard threshold shift, it is the obligation of the company to take immediate responsive action. The first action is, of course, informing (in writing) the affected person. The second action is implementing "appropriate" correction. Just what constitutes appropriate corrective action is certainly highly problematic because it encompasses not only regulatory mandates, but ethical and moral considerations as well—most of which are well beyond contemporary regulatory jurisdiction.

In the case where a standard threshold shift is attributed to or aggravated by workplace noise, American OSHA regulations are clear about several required corrective actions, including:

- other personnel who work in a similar workplace situation as that by the person who experienced the standard threshold shift and who do not use hearing protectors will be fitted with hearing protectors, trained in their use and care, and required to use them

- other personnel who work in a workplace situation similar to that of the person who experienced the standard threshold shift and who do use hearing protectors will be refitted and retrained in the use of hearing protectors and, if necessary, provided with protectors offering greater noise attenuation
- the person affected by the work-related standard threshold shift will be referred to a clinical audiological evaluation or otological examination

These regulations, however, do not define those actions to be taken with regard to the future needs of an employee who has suffered work-related hearing impairment, or of the employee who has suffered hearing impairment that, while detected by means of the corporate audiometric testing program, is not caused or aggravated by workplace noise. In reality, the former will be decided by the legalities of corporate health plans or by formal litigation; the latter, ignored—though with due corporate regard for the real potential for subsequent litigation.

Regulatory authority ultimately rests, after all, upon social convention. Despite recent and rather dramatic instances of the public's willingness to interject changing social values into day-to-day corporate decision-making, even the most demanding of workplace regulations finally relies upon the accessibility of employees to more public fora than the board room, including legislatures and the courts. During this long protracted readjustment of traditional corporate practice and regulatory constraint to social dialectics, the safety officer must be pointedly reminded of a cardinal rule: compliance with the requisite actions defined by a regulatory bureaucracy does not exhaust the range of legal, ethical, or moral responsibilities that, in any particular situation, may emerge as even more demanding and infinitely more authoritative.

HEARING PROTECTORS AND NOISE ATTENUATION

Wherever engineering and managerial strategies do not reduce the exposure of employees below the action level, the safety officer must ensure that personnel are provided with hearing protectors.

There are four basic types of earplugs, each having certain advantages and limitations, especially with regard to personal comfort level:

1. Enclosure: helmet type protection, typically providing attenuation of 35 dB at <1000 Hz and 50 dB at >1000 Hz; while highly effective for attenuating sound conducted through air, not very effective for attenuating sound conducted through bone or body; relatively bulky and uncomfortable

for most work situations; generally used where both hearing and head protection are required.

2. Aural insert (earplug): most commonly used type of protector in industry; inserted into the ear to plug the ear canal; provides attenuation of up to 25 dB at <1000 Hz and 35 dB at >1000 Hz, with common attenuations in the workplace of 5–15 dB and 15–25 dB, respectively; three different types commonly available:

    A. Formable earplug: designed to be discarded after one-time use; made of expandable foams, glass fiber, wax impregnated cotton, Swedish wool, or mineral-down; degree of attenuation depends on snugness of fit

    B. Custom molded earplug: designed to fit an individual's ear; changes in ear canal and drying of the mold material can detract from effectiveness

    C. Premolded earplug: made of soft silicone, rubber or plastic; fit generic shapes of ear canals; various modifications for particular industrial settings, including modifications for differential attenuations at different frequencies and for various combinations of continuous or impact noise; some models developed for specific occupational groups (e.g., musicians).

3. Canal cap (semi- and supraaural): used to seal external opening of the ear canal (as opposed to plugging the ear canal); held in place by band or other head suspension device; range of attenuation comparable to that by earplug; ideal for intermittent use.

4. Earmuff (circumaural device): domed cup covering the entire external ear; can provide up to 35 dB attenuation at <1000 Hz and 45 dB at higher frequencies, but with many workplace attenuations reaching only 10–12 dB; may be uncomfortable due to slight pressure applied to side of head.

In the United States, specific requirements for hearing protectors and standards for determining the degree of noise attenuation offered by different types of protectors are provided by 29 CFR 1910.95 (i) and (j). Basically, these regulations require that affected employees wear protectors that attenuate exposure at least to an 8-hr TWA of 90 dB or, in the case of any employee who has experienced a standard threshold shift, at least 85 dB. While these regulations do not specifically address contractors or other persons who may be on company premises (e.g., visitors, governmental inspectors), many companies establish clearly marked zones within the workplace where the wearing of hearing protectors is required by all persons who enter, regardless of status.

While the regulations do require that the adequacy of hearing protectors be reevaluated whenever workplace noise increases to a potentially dangerous level, they do not provide practical criteria for making that determination. It is therefore recommended that the safety officer establish such criteria, which might reasonably include:

- the installation of new machines and equipment of substantially different design or function from machines and equipment that have already been evaluated with respect to the requirements of the HCP
- changes in production schedules or techniques that may result in different levels of combined workplace noise
- changes in personnel work assignments that may result in different levels of cumulative noise experienced by those personnel
- initiation of on-site construction or refurbishment that may introduce new sources of noise into the workplace environment

EMPLOYEE TRAINING

The HCP must contain detailed information regarding the mandatory annual training of affected personnel. Specifically, training must address at the least the following types of information:

- the effects of noise on hearing
- the purpose of hearing protectors, the advantages, disadvantages, and attenuation of various types of protectors, and instructions for selecting, fitting, using, and maintaining them
- the purpose of audiometric testing and an explanation of test procedures

It is particularly important to stress company policies regarding the mandatory use of hearing protection. In many companies, employees are often confused about what is mandatory and what is optional in terms of various types of protective clothing and equipment. The safety officer must therefore ensure that affected personnel fully understand that they must wear hearing protectors—that, except for possible choices from among various types and styles that provide the same required minimum protection while at the same time differences in personal comfort level, there is no option. In this regard, it is strongly recommended that training also include a thorough explanation of personnel actions that will be taken in cases where affected employees disregard company policy. All employees should also understand their role in ensuring that contractors and other plant visitors comply with the provisions of the HCP.

RECORD KEEPING

In the United States, record-keeping practices related to workplace health and safety must conform to the provisions of 29 CFR 1910.20 as specified in individual health and safety regulations. Under 29 CFR 1910.95, all records related to ambient noise monitoring and audiometric tests, including monitoring data and calibration data, are pertinent. A key provision is that all such records be provided upon request to employees, former employees, and any representative designated by the individual employee as well as to appropriate regulatory authority.

Given the increasingly expanded, legally mandated accessibility of employees to corporate records related to their health and safety, and given the direct relevance of such records to potential litigation, the safety officer is well advised to exercise the most meticulous care with regard to the management of records. Perhaps the most useful advice is to consider regulatory requirements regarding the types of information to be retained as minimal. For example, while there is no specific regulatory requirement in 29 CFR 1910.95 to maintain a written record of the proceedings of a preliminary meeting between the safety officer and the company's contracted consultant for ambient monitoring, there are many circumstances that might eventually develop in which such a record may become (for medical or legal reasons) precisely relevant and utterly important. Anecdotal evidence to the contrary, in regard to human health and legal litigation there is no such thing as too much documentation.

CHAPTER 12

HAZARDOUS WASTE MANAGEMENT

BACKGROUND

There is no issue, either from a national or an international perspective, that better represents the need for a broadly comprehensive and highly integrative management of human health and environmental quality than the issue of hazardous waste. At the nexus between environmental and social dynamics, between ecological and economic productivity, and between the health and well-being of current and future human populations, the concern for managing hazardous wastes has dominated much of the American environmental legislative agenda over the past quarter century and can be expected to continue to profoundly influence international politics, trade, and law.

Concurrent both then and now with ongoing legislative efforts related to water and air quality, the first major Federal effort to manage hazardous waste was taken in 1976 with congressional enactment of the Resource Conservation and Recovery Act (RCRA)—an act that has generally come to be known as the "hazardous waste act" but which, in reality, is a "solid waste act" that broadly encompasses not only hazardous wastes but all solid wastes.

The focus of hazardous waste management under RCRA is the so-called "cradle-to-grave" management of waste generated by existing facilities during ongoing production activities. Four years after the enactment of RCRA, Congress expanded the management of hazardous wastes by enacting the Comprehensive Environmental Response, Compensation and Liability Act (CERCLA). Widely known as "Superfund," this act focuses on the management of hazardous wastes previously disposed, most often by now defunct companies.

Both RCRA and CERCLA underscore national intent to establish and enforce the effective management of human health and safety, including the health and safety of not only company employees who may become exposed to hazardous wastes as a result of routine and emergency workplace operations, but also of the larger community.

In the context of RCRA, practices and procedures related to actual and potential emergencies must be addressed in a written "contingency plan" or "spill control plan." With regard to both RCRA and CERCLA, health and safety precautions for *emergency responders* are subject to the requirements of 29 CFR 1910.120. Emergency response (including 29 CFR 1910.120), which is discussed in detail in Chapter 13, is today a rapidly developing specialty that must be inclusive of a wide range of regulatory and corporate managerial issues. Here the focus is on those aspects of the routine day-to-day management of hazardous wastes that are of particular relevance to workplace health and safety.

RESPONSIBILITY

Most companies give overall responsibility for hazardous waste management to a person designated as the hazardous waste manager (HWM) or, variously, the "hazardous waste coordinator" or "hazardous waste engineer." This may or may not be the same person designated as the emergency response coordinator (ERC), who has specific responsibilities under the RCRA Contingency Plan that must be implemented in an actual or potential emergency.

Despite regulatory differences due to the different enabling legislation of various countries and, in the United States, of those states granted *primacy* under the Federal RCRA (i.e., the right of a state to enforce a federal law within that state), important generic regulatory compliance responsibilities of the HWM typically include:

- Fulfillment of all hazardous waste licensing or permit requirements
- Identification of specific hazardous wastes generated and/or handled
- Proper labeling, marking, and/or placarding of hazardous waste containers
- Development and implementation of all policies, procedures and practices regarding the collection, storage, transportation, and disposal of hazardous wastes
- Management of all hazardous waste manifests and other documents pertinent to the management of hazardous wastes
- Design and implementation of a personnel training program
- Design and implementation of a hazardous waste contingency program

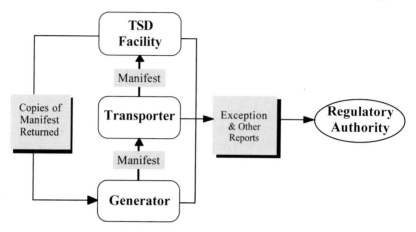

FIGURE 12.1   Overview of the "cradle-to-grave" management of hazardous waste. Manifests and other reporting requirements lay down a "paper trail" for the movement of hazardous wastes from the point of generation to their final disposal. An essential feature of this management system is the licensing (or permitting) of generators, transporters, and treatment/storage/disposal (TSD) facilities.

While the above responsibilities reflect basic tasks identified in RCRA and similar legislation in other countries, the HWC is today increasingly likely to have additional responsibilities that reflect the growing recognition of even broader implications of modern hazardous waste management, especially with regard to (a) potential intrusion into corporate property of hazardous wastes produced by external sources, (b) acquisition of new property that may be contaminated with hazardous wastes, (c) potential contamination of air, water, and soil resources not only through corporate operations, but also structural or other materials (e.g., asbestos insulation, materials impregnated with toxic paints or preservatives), and (d) the potential liabilities associated with the failure to minimize the generation of hazardous wastes. The first three of these concerns have historically been the province of property management; the last, of operations planning.

Among regulatory compliance, property management and operations planning tasks are certain tasks that, because of their complexity and their direct impact on worker health and safety, deserve particular emphasis.

SELECTED REGULATORY COMPLIANCE TASKS

As shown in Figure 12.1, RCRA's cradle-to-grave approach to managing those hazardous wastes derived from ongoing corporate operations requires the coordinated control of licensed (or permitted) generators, transporters, and treatment–storage–disposal (TSD) facilities. This control is basically accomplished by means of the *hazardous waste manifest* (or shipping paper, bill of laden) on which the generator of the waste specifies (among other things) the type and amount of waste, the transporter who accepts the waste for transportation, and the TSD facility to which the waste is ultimately transported for final treatment or disposal. Records of copies of manifests kept by generators, transporters, and TSD facilities as well as by the responsible governmental authority (e.g., U.S. Environmental Protection Agency or, in states granted primacy, state authority), and prescribed manifest return and reporting requirements (including TSD confirmation of waste receipt, annual or biannual summary activity reports, *exception reports*) provide the essential "paper-trail" that ensures the proper flow of hazardous waste from the generator's "cradle" to the TSD facility's "grave."

Because the hazardous waste manifest represents a tightly interlocked system of licensing, documenting, and reporting requirements that impose significant legal liability, much of the effort of the HWC is devoted to the in-plant management of manifests. While the importance of giving meticulous attention to manifests cannot be overstressed, other tasks are of at least equal if not more immediate importance to the health and safety of company employees and the surrounding community.

Identification of Hazardous Wastes

The responsibility for deciding which company wastes are legally hazardous wastes and therefore subject to regulatory control is solely that of the company. Regulations provide protocols for making that determination. Under RCRA, for example, a waste may be determined to be subject to RCRA because it (a) is listed in the regulations by name (e.g., benzene) or general source (e.g., still bottoms) or (b) has one or more hazardous characteristics, including *ignitability* (flash point $< 140°F$), *corrosivity* (pH ≤ 2 or ≥ 12.5), *reactivity* (explosive, produces toxic gases when mixed with water or acid), and *toxicity* (when subjected to standardized leachate tests, waste releases chemical species and concentrations as specified in the regulations).

Compliance with identification requirements presumes that the HWC has performed a comprehensive in-plant survey (or audit) of all potential wastes. In the modern corporation that recognizes the need for an integrated HSE approach to business management, such a survey is, in fact, but one aspect of a comprehensive chemical safety audit (Chapters 4, 5, and 6). Under no circumstance should the HWC consider only those wastes defined by plant production processes. Potential hazardous wastes certainly include operational wastes, but they also include by-product wastes as well as wastes derived from other sources, such as accidental spills of virgin materials and discarded or off-spec materials.

The HWC is reminded that the mere absence of a waste's name in a RCRA list (or of the names of its constituents), does not preclude the waste from being a regulated hazardous waste. It may, after all, be listed by generic source or because it meets a RCRA-defined hazardous characteristic. Unfortunately, many HWC rely upon the opinion of vendors as to whether or not a particular material may qualify as a hazardous waste—a practice that in no way whatsoever abrogates corporate responsibility for determining the regulatory status of the material. Where a material is not listed either by name or source, and where its hazardous characteristics cannot be determined solely on the basis of standard technical or scientific literature, the HWC should submit the material to a certified analytical laboratory for testing and subsequent determination. In such a case, the HWC is advised to ensure that the so-called "certified laboratory" is specifically certified to perform the RCRA-specified tests.

The HWC is also reminded that, historically, the determination of the regulatory status of a waste under RCRA is totally independent of the concentration of any hazardous ingredient—a practice that reflects the persistently influential adage, "Dilution is not the solution to pollution."

In-Plant Labeling

U.S. EPA requirements for the labeling of hazardous waste containers under RCRA are quite different from labeling requirements of other chemical containers under OSHA regulations, and both RCRA and OSHA in-plant labeling requirements differ from U.S. Department of Transportation (DOT) requirements for chemical containers in public transport. For example, it may be necessary to describe precisely the same liquid using either:

- a single hazard class, such as "flammable liquid" (DOT), or
- the chemical name, such as "Benzene," followed by the full range of potential hazards, including physical and health hazards, routes of entry, and target organs (OSHA), or
- the proper shipping name of the hazardous waste, such as "Waste Flammable Liquid; Benzene" (EPA)

Given the ubiquity of the computer, the HWC is well advised to coordinate with the corporate safety officer or other personnel having other regulatory responsibility (e.g., hazard communication, laboratory hygiene) to ensure that a computerized chemical inventory contains sufficiently diverse algorithms to meet the labeling requirements (including both format and informational requirements) of different regulations that apply to the same chemical material.

Development of Written SOPs

Written SOPs should specify all actions that personnel should perform to ensure the safe handling and storage of any hazardous waste. As shown in Table 12.1, these actions include (a) any preparatory steps to be taken prior to initiating a particular activity, (b) the use of personal protective clothing and equipment, (c) and operational standards that may apply to various steps or stages of the activity.

Ideally located in the immediate area in which the activity is to be performed, such SOPs are today most directly accessible through computer terminals, the use of which is often required as a part of the work authorization process. This approach also provides the safety officer and operational managers a direct means (i.e., through monitoring of employee use of computer files) of exerting appropriate quality or oversight control of all activities related to the handling of hazardous wastes.

As shown in Table 12.1, SOPs should give particular emphasis to directions directly pertinent to the behavior of personnel. Behavioral commands such as "wear," "open," and "close" are infinitely more useful than commands such as "ensure," "understand," and "exercise appropriate care."

It must be understood that the investment of time regarding the development of effective SOPs is significant, requiring the close coordination of the HWC with operational supervisors and personnel who are most knowledgeable about the practical aspects of job tasks. Draft SOPs should be shop tested thoroughly before they are finalized.

In all instances, the development of a useful SOP requires detailed consideration of relevant technical information and data that directly relates to health and safety. Examples of such information and data include:

- the compatibility of different hazardous wastes, which determines which hazardous wastes may be mixed without the risk of explosion, the production of toxic gases, or other dangerous reactions
- physical factors that influence the reactivity of individual hazardous wastes, including potential reaction to changes in pressure, temperature, physical shock, the intensity of light, and electrical potential
- the capacities and limitations of protective clothing and equipment, including the use of protective tools such as nonsparking, insulated, and electrical grounding devices

Under no circumstance should the HWC rely solely on information obtained from MSDSs or the nondocumented advice given by materials vendors; the technical information base pertaining to such matters is extensive, easily available through commercial sources, and also available in both computerized and printed format at little cost. Such items as chemical compatibility charts, texts and matrices on physical–chemical factors

TABLE 12.1 Example of an Industrial Standard Operating Procedure Regarding the Handling of a Hazardous Waste Acid

---

	SOP 112.81
Global Enterprises, Inc	Transfer Waste Acid to Storage Tanks
	Page 1 of 4

The following conditions must be met prior to undertaking any transfer of waste acid to storage tanks:

- Only the Treatment Facility Operator may perform the transfer
- Acid to be transferred must be cooled to 70° or less prior to transfer
- There must be enough space in the waste acid storage tank to accommodate the entire amount of acid plus 10%
- Air agitation pump in acid tank and acid recirculation pump must be turned off
- Transfer ejector discharge valve must be in open position

Wear →	Acid resistant, steel-toed boots, acid resistant jacket and trousers (or overalls), acid resistant gloves, face shield and attaching helmet, and full face piece respirator with acid gas cartridge. All items are located in 'AT Locker'.
Test →	Safety shower, eye wash, and telephone at signed transfer area
Inspect →	All equipment and piping continually throughout transfer process for leaks, particularly pipelines passing overhead to the outside
Monitor →	• Level in Waste Acid Storage Tank • Temperature of discharge nozzle to storage tank
Place →	Transfer ejector suction hose inlet in water rinse tank nearest to the waste acid
Open →	Manual steam valve to ejector, checking that regulated pressure is 55 to 60 psi; then start ejector

---

governing chemical reactivity, and catalogs of protective clothing and equipment should be considered as standard technical references in any modern corporation.

Storage of Wastes

Written SOPs regarding the storage of wastes are particularly important because both long- and short-term storage areas present particularly high health and safety risks.

In addition to the RCRA standards for storage areas, including the *main accumulation area*, which may be used for the long-term storage of hazardous wastes (i.e., up to 90 or 180 days for large and small quantity generators, respectively), and *satellite accumulation areas*, which may be located in the immediate area in which the waste is generated and used only for short-term storage (e.g., up to 3 days for a maximum of 55 gallons of nonacutely hazardous waste), SOPs should include due consideration of the following issues:

1. The mixing of various wastes in one container (*waste consolidation*) offers significant savings in disposal costs compared with the disposal of many small containers of individual wastes. However, mixing different wastes always carries the risks associated with chemical incompatibility, either through oversight or other human error. It is advisable that the HWC (a) not allow any mixing of wastes to be performed in satellite accumulation areas and (b) allow mixing in the main accumulation area only by specified personnel who must follow a detailed written protocol.

2. Except where provided with state-of-art protection (including continuous external ventilation, temperature control, spill containment, blowout external wall panels, spark-proof electrical system, electrical grounding, automatic fire suppression system, and automatic monitoring of chemical vapors), it is advisable that the main accumulation area be located outside major facility buildings. Many moderately priced modular sheds specifically designed for the storage of hazardous waste are available. The HWC should coordinate with the local fire chief before selecting and locating an appropriate model. Whether the main accumulation area is located inside or external to a facility building, access by company personnel should be stringently controlled, and all practicable measures should be taken to deny access to nonauthorized persons.

3. Satellite accumulation areas should provide for the immediate containment of spills and leaks and protect against seepage of hazardous waste into pervious floors. The areas should be completely accessible at all times, with proper emergency equipment (e.g., fire extinguisher) immediately available. The location should also ensure that the waste is compatible with ambient conditions. For example, under no circumstance should a water-reactive waste be stored in a sprinklered area or where water vapors or mists are generated by production processes or housekeeping activities. Similarly, flammable wastes having high vapor density should not be stored in an area where there are subfloor electrical conduits.

Personnel Training

In addition to the training of emergency response personnel, the HWC must evaluate the training needs of all company personnel. It is useful to distinguish between "broad" and "special" training needs among plant personnel; broad needs reflect required levels of awareness of hazardous waste policies and procedures, and special needs, those skills that individuals who have specific responsibilities for hazardous waste must demonstrate. Training should not be targeted to job titles (e.g., department managers and supervisors, office staff, technicians, and laborers) except as such job titles denote specific responsibility for the management of hazardous wastes. In this regard, the HWC must remember that a key requirement of RCRA is written job descriptions of personnel having responsibilities for hazardous waste. This provision, too often overlooked or purposely ignored, is the only logical basis for implementing an effective, performance-based training program.

Contaminated Property

While the responsibility of the HWC has historically been limited to concerns regarding the in-plant production of hazardous wastes, the knowledge and experience of the HWC is also directly relevant to corporate planning regarding the acquisition of new property that may, in fact, already be contaminated with hazardous chemicals. In the United States, the provisions of CERCLA have forced corporations to give special attention to the potential liabilities that might be associated with the acquisition of potentially contaminated property. In many instances, this has resulted not only in the increased use of consultants who specialize in the investigation of contaminated property but also in a greatly expanded liaison among the corporate safety officer, the hazardous waste coordinator, and external consultants. Such liaison becomes important not only in protecting the corporation from legal risks and its employees from health and safety risks associated with the acquisition of contaminated property, but also in taking proactive steps to ensure that present corporate property does not become, in the future, a contaminated site.

Various techniques are available for assessing the potential chemical contamination of property. However, depending on the size of the property, some of these techniques may not be appropriate. Moreover, prior to the actual legal acquisition of property, very real constraints exist on what can actually be accomplished in terms of site evaluation and analytical testing. Basically, the typical assessment process consists of (a) a site inspection, (b) a background records search, and (c) a subsurface investigation.

Site Inspection

A preliminary site inspection is a visual examination of the property to identify any possible structures, activities, features, or conditions that might indicate historical or possibly future releases of chemicals. The inspection should be carried out by persons who are familiar with the local area in terms of land use, types of industry, and agricultural practices. At least one member of the inspection team should be a chemical health and safety officer specifically trained in the recognition of chemical hazards.

During the inspection, particular attention should be given to the following:

- present and historical usage of the site
- structures, including purpose and type of construction, with special regard for construction materials that present special hazards (e.g., lead paint, asbestos)
- above- and below-ground storage areas possibly used for chemical storage, including tanks (and associated piping), drums, sheds, and stockpiles
- cesspools and sanitary tanks that might contain hazardous chemicals in addition to sewage
- ditches, storm drains, catch basins, and floor drains
- paved surfaces (bitumen and concrete) that may later have to be sounded to ensure that they are not hiding pits, tanks, and pipes containing hazardous chemicals
- surface water supplies, including open water and wetland areas that might serve as receiving systems for land runoff carrying hazardous chemicals
- conditions of abutting properties, including structures and activities that could result in the release of chemicals (e.g., spraying of pesticides, leaking underground tanks)
- hydrologic gradients in the general area, and land use patterns of up- and downgradient properties
- prevailing wind patterns in the general area, and land use patterns of up- and downwind properties
- visual or other evidence (e.g., smells) of previous releases of chemicals, including round stains, obvious water pollution (e.g., oil scums), stressed vegetation, and trash piles containing pails or other possible chemical containers or contaminated materials, including old pipes, construction debris, and tires

- records associated with on-site operation of current facilities, including permits, waste disposal records, chemical inventories, and MSDSs

In pursuit of this information, the best practice is to begin a site inspection only after a careful review of aerial photographs and topographic and geological maps. Conversing with local residents who are likely to have a much better appreciation of local problems that might be related to the release of hazardous chemicals into the environment is also a good idea.

Background Records Search

Having conducted a preliminary site inspection, the assessment team should undertake a thorough search of records that might indicate past releases of chemicals that might have contaminated the property. The sources of records of interest will vary, of course, with the particular legal jurisdiction. Examples of the types of information and potential sources that are generally useful include:

- underground storage tank registration (e.g., local fire department, town or city authorities)
- permits for sewage discharge (e.g., sewer authority, department of public works)
- historical ownership of property (local assessor's office, town clerk)
- water table and artesian wells in general vicinity (local water department or company, department of public works)
- wetland and other natural resources that might have been affected by earlier releases (e.g., local conservation commission, department of environmental protection, police and fire department)
- reported releases (police and fire department, environmental authority, local emergency response company or agency)
- water quality and other reports, including ambient quality of resources (department of environmental protection, water resources and wildlife regulatory authorities)

Subsurface Investigation

Conducting a subsurface investigation of property prior to purchase is difficult if not actually impossible. However, the importance of a subsurface investigation cannot be overemphasized and every effort should be made to implement one at least as a condition of purchase.

No subsurface investigation should be undertaken until the chemical health and safety officer has devised a comprehensive site safety plan and all field personnel have been trained in its proper implementation, the proper use of field monitors (e.g., oxygen meter, combustion meter, organic vapor detector) and personal protective clothing and equipment. Particularly hazardous conditions noted in the field—such as drums of unknown chemicals, flammable storage sheds, and smells of organic vapors—should be reported immediately to local safety and health officials. All field work should be suspended until appropriate remedial action has been completed.

Techniques typically employed during a subsurface investigation include:

1. Manual digging/drilling: use of shovel and/or auger to determine depth of soil staining; investigate suspicious soils; take limited depth samples for chemical analysis
2. Backhoe trenching: to expose soil profiles to a depth of 10–12 feet; collect soil samples; identify refuse and other burials
3. Drilling: techniques that do not use drilling fluids are to be preferred; obtain deep soil samples for subsequent laboratory analysis; establish subsurface stratigraphy; establish wells that can be used to monitor up- and downgradient water quality for documenting on-site water soluble soil contaminants
4. Geophysical investigatory techniques: to locate buried tanks and pipes
5. Electronic detection of volatile gases: used in combination with manual digging, backhoe trenching, and/or drilling

Of course, there are limitations associated with each technique. For example, manual digging, backhoe trenching, and drilling cannot be applied to an entire property. These methods should be used only when there is reason to suspect that a particular location might be contaminated. Drilling is most often employed to determine basic groundwater flow patterns and to establish a relatively small number of water quality monitoring wells, not to identify a particular source of contamination, except as part of an investigation of plume flow. It should be noted that companies increasingly establish monitoring wells at the periphery of corporate property as a means of detecting incursions of contaminated groundwater from external sources.

All samples collected for subsequent laboratory analysis should be collected, preserved, and stored according to specific written directions supplied by the laboratory. Parameters to be tested in soil and water samples should minimally include those designated by legal authority as directly relevant to the determination of hazardous wastes and regulated priority pollutants. These substances typically include volatile organics (including halogenated solvents), base/neutral acid extractables (such as polynuclear aromatic hydrocarbons, phthalate esters, semivolatile aromatic compounds, and phenolic compounds), pesticides and polychlorinated biphenyls, and inorganic compounds (such as heavy metals and cyanides).

A particular problem associated with property acquisition is the demolition of structures on acquired property. Ordinarily, the removal of structures and hauling away of wastes is left, all other things being equal, to the lowest bidder. However, the assessment team should evaluate the demolition process as potentially generating a regulated hazardous waste, a situation that would require specifically trained and licensed personnel to remove and properly dispose of demolition wastes.

After all, finding hazardous chemicals stored behind bricked-up walls or under concrete floors of abandoned industrial buildings is not a particularly uncommon event. Asbestos may be included in various components of the structure or its appurtenances. Lead paint may cover wooden surfaces. Creosote may saturate posts and beams. Oils may clog cellar soils. Heavy metals and a wide variety of organic solvents may remain in cesspools and sanitary drains or be absorbed into metal and concrete pipes.

Waste Minimization

Under the U.S. Hazardous and Solid Waste Amendments of 1984, each generator of hazardous waste must certify that, in its treatment, storage and disposal of hazardous waste, the company has taken every practicable measure to minimize any present and future threat to human health and the environment. This certification is typically imprinted on each hazardous waste manifest. Unfortunately, even after a dozen years, many generators complete this certification without giving it any substantive attention.

The management of hazardous waste does not begin and end with compliance with the hazard waste manifest system. Hazardous waste management must always presume a good-faith effort to minimize the generation of hazardous waste. Waste minimization, which is also variously called "waste reduction," "pollution prevention," or "green production," has somewhat different meanings according to different regulatory authority, but typically includes the following categorical types of approaches to inventory management, modification of production processes, the reduction of waste volume, and resource recovery:

1. Chemical substitution: the substitution of a non (or less)-hazardous chemical input to a production process for a hazardous chemical; this approach recognizes that such a substitution may not be possible, but requires a methodical assessment of the state-of-art and ongoing research and development

2. Product reformulation: the reformulation of a product so that it requires less of a hazardous raw material to produce it; in many instances, a product is formulated simply on the basis of historical precedent, without

due consideration of changes that can be made to reduce the concentration of a hazardous constituent either in the final product or in a catalyst or by-product of the production process

3. Efficiency improvement: a change in the production process so that it uses necessary hazardous substances more efficiently; in some cases, this might involve reengineering a production process or it might simply involve better management of operational habits or practices

4. In-process recycling: recycling a hazardous material directly into the production process to reduce final volume or otherwise reduce the total amount of hazardous material needed as feedstock; recycling that is carried on external to the production process that created it is not generally considered waste minimization because such recycling does not reduce the total amount of hazardous waste produced and, in some instances, may even result in an increase

5. Housekeeping: those practices specifically implemented to reduce the amount of hazardous waste ultimately released to the work or ambient environment, including practices regarding the detection and control of fugitive emissions, spills and leaks

In some legal jurisdictions (e.g., some states in the United States), waste minimization is a key objective of legislation that is generally described as *toxics use reduction* legislation, which requires the submission to regulatory authority of written plans demonstrating how a company intends to achieve targeted reductions in the use of specifically identified hazardous substances, either as inputs to or outputs from the production process or even ancillary corporate operations. Whether through the increasing efforts of the U.S. EPA to enforce the broad policy objectives of RCRA or through state (or even Federal) "toxics use reduction" legislation, the HWC is strongly advised that waste minimization is rapidly becoming a major aspect of hazardous waste management and already demands serious corporate attention.

OSHA SUBPART Z STANDARDS

In many instances, the HWC is tempted to focus so intently on RCRA regulations as to overlook the requirements of 29 CFR 1910, subpart Z, which includes specific requirements regarding over two dozen chemical substances, including generic categories (e.g., air contaminants, coal tar pitch volatiles) as well as individual chemical species (e.g., 4-nitrobiphenyl; benzidine; acrylonitrile). The HWC (or safety officer) employed by a transporter or TSD facility must recognize that a hazardous waste manifest prepared by the generator in full compliance with RCRA does not contain sufficient information to assure compliance with the limits and controls imposed by 29 CFR 1910, subpart Z. The transporter or TSD HWC should therefore request additional information about the generator's waste regarding subpart Z constituents. The prudent generator HWC will integrate subpart Z requirements with the identification of hazardous waste constituents. All SOPs regarding the in-plant handling and ambient monitoring of hazardous wastes containing such constituents should be in full compliance with subpart Z.

RISKS ASSOCIATED WITH RCRA EXEMPTED MATERIALS

RCRA as well as some comparable enabling legislation in other countries specifically exempts certain materials, including domestic sewage and any mixture of domestic sewage and other waste that passes through a sewer system to a publicly owned treatment works (POTW). In the industrial setting, such mixtures of sewage and "other waste" can be generated from the flow of workplace waste through floor drains into a plant's sewer pipes.

In many instances, POTWs enforce contractual rules with industry that preclude industrial discharge containing any RCRA hazardous waste; also, *industrial pretreatment regulations* (under the Clean Water Act, CWA) are increasingly effective in preventing the industrial discharge of RCRA or other regulated chemicals through POTW-treated sewage.

However, depending upon specific contractual requirements of POTWs and regulatory requirements regarding industrial pretreatment of sewer discharge, POTW employees are subject to exposure to dangerous chemicals in industrial waste streams, and companies that generate these waste streams are consequently at risk of lawsuits initiated by affected POTW employees.

Another example of workers who might be adversely affected by sewage containing hazardous or toxic materials and who might also be the source of corporate legal risk are those employees or contractors who might be required to conduct in-plant maintenance of sewer pipes and connections. At special risk are those who become exposed to hazardous fumes and dusts or absorb toxic chemicals directly through skin contact, for example, through welding or cutting pipes that might concentrate hazardous chemicals out of the sewage into pipe linings, or through the excavation of soils contaminated by leaking pipes.

In light of this very common threat of exposure to hazardous chemicals and of litigation, the HWC is advised to take all practical steps to ensure that no industrial waste inadvertently enters into the plant's sewer disposal system. This typically involves at least the covering or plugging of floor drains and, where combined sewers are used, the plugging of yard drains and conduits that might receive runoff containing industrial chemicals (e.g., yard drains in the vicinity of loading docks and chemical storage areas).

GENERATOR STATUS

From the beginning, RCRA provided different requirements for the large quantity generator and small quantity generator, distinguished from each other by the total volume of hazardous waste produced monthly. Various states, granted primacy under RCRA, have also developed additional distinctions among generators, such as:

- Large quantity generator (LQG): generates more than 1000 kg (2200 lbs.) of hazardous waste in 1 month; once the first 1000 kg has been accumulated, the waste must be shipped within 90 days; there is no limit to the amount of hazardous waste that can be accumulated
- Small quantity generator (SQG): generates less than 1000 kg of hazardous waste in 1 month and/or less than 1 kg of "acutely hazardous waste" (as listed by regulation)
- Very small quantity generator (VSQG): generates less than 100 kg of hazardous waste in 1 month and generates no acutely hazardous waste

Originally, the regulatory requirements for the SQG were quite minimal; however, in 1986, the U.S. EPA promulgated regulations for the SQG that made them essentially comparable to regulations for the LQG, and some states (e.g., California) implemented legislation specifically requiring all generators, regardless of status based on the volume of waste production, to comply with all hazardous waste regulations.

Where distinctions among generators are legally permitted on the basis of waste volume, many companies that are essentially borderline with regard to one or another distinction opt for what they consider to be the less stringent requirement. This is sometimes done by conveniently overlooking certain wastes, which is a flagrant flouting of regulations, but it is also often accomplished by making straightforward and eminently legal decisions regarding various business options that influence the volume of waste generated, such as the decision to introduce a new production line.

In either case, the HWC is reminded of a basic principle that is applicable not only to hazardous waste regulations, but to all regulations that influence workplace health and safety: regulations designed to minimize the health and safety of workers and to protect environmental quality also serve to lessen the risk of corporate liability. To opt, where possible, for the lesser of regulatory stringency may certainly result in immediate economic benefits, but it also increases the probability of significant longer-range liabilities that are inclusive of personal as well as corporate economic and legal risks.

GENERATOR INSPECTION OF TRANSPORTER AND TSD FACILITIES

Perhaps the most practical rule governing a generator's management of hazardous waste is: "Once you generate a hazardous waste, it is yours forever." Generators must understand that this rule applies even after a waste has been disposed of by a licensed TSD facility. Responsibility for the waste always belongs to the generator; it cannot be given away or sold or otherwise contracted to anyone else.

Because any failure of the transporter or TSD facility that accepts a generator's waste imposes a legal liability on not only that transporter or TSD facility but also the generator, the prudent generator must exercise quality control over the activities of the transporter and TSD facility. This is usually accomplished by the generator conducting at least an annual site audit of transporter and TSD facilities. During this audit, the generator reviews all aspects of actual operations, with particular regard to specific policies and procedures governing both normal operations and emergencies.

In addition to the site visit, the HWC is also advised to contact local legal authorities (e.g., department of environmental protection, department of public health, fire department) to review any incident reports or complaints regarding transporter or TSD operations. Where possible, it is also a good idea to confer with other corporate clients of the transporter and TSD facility regarding their experience and concerns.

The HWC should include all findings in a written evaluation of the transporter and TSD facility, along with a clear assessment of the reasons to continue or terminate the professional services of the transporter or TSD facility. The HWC is reminded that this document may become a key document in future legal proceedings in which the generator may find it necessary to defend itself for having selected a contractor who subsequently demonstrates negligence or incompetence or otherwise incurs regulatory, civil, or even criminal liability.

CHAPTER 13

EMERGENCY RESPONSE

BACKGROUND

Emergency response planning is rapidly becoming an integral component of routine corporate management that, while directly influenced by a variety of specific regulations at all levels of government, is also often influenced by nonregulatory considerations, including obligations imposed by corporate insurance policies, the demands of both *ad hoc* and formal in-plant safety committees, and the widespread concern regarding terrorist acts of groups and individuals.

In the United States, the primary Federal influence on corporate emergency response planning is through that legislation governing the corporate generation of hazardous waste (RCRA) and activities associated with uncontrolled hazardous waste sites (CERCLA and related "Superfund" legislation, especially Title I of the Superfund Amendments and Reauthorization Act [SARA]), although other legislation and regulations also establish emergency response requirements, including the Clean Water Act (CWA), the Hazardous Material Transportation Act (HMTA), and the Chemical Process Safety Regulations (29 CFR 1910.119).

With respect to the health and safety of workers involved in emergency response, the controlling baseline regulations are 29 CFR 1910.120 (Hazardous Waste Operations and Emergency Response) and 29 CFR 1910.38 (Employee Emergency Plans), which contain appropriate cross-references to additional regulations (e.g., respiratory protection, alarm systems, eye and foot protection, etc.).

Under 29 CFR 1910.120, a written *emergency response plan* must describe how an actual emergency will be handled to minimize risks to three groups of personnel:

1. employees engaged in cleanups at uncontrolled hazardous waste sites

2. employees engaged in routine operations and corrective actions at RCRA facilities
3. employees engaged in emergency response without regard to location

Where the employer does not allow employees to respond to an emergency in any manner except by evacuating premises, the employer must develop a written *emergency action plan*, which (in compliance with 29 CFR 1910.39) includes the following minimum elements:

- emergency escape procedures and routes
- procedures to be followed by employees who remain to operate critical plant operations before they evacuate
- procedures to account for all employees after emergency evacuation has been completed
- rescue and medical duties for those employees who are to perform them
- the preferred means of reporting fires and other emergencies
- names or job titles of persons or departments who can be contacted for further information or explanations of duties associated with emergency response

Depending on relevant regulatory requirements, the overall in-plant responsibility for emergency response planning and implementation may be assigned to the "primary emergency response coordinator" (e.g., under RCRA regulations), the "Site Safety and Health Supervisor" (e.g., under 29 CFR 1910.120), or to any number of variously titled personnel having specialized knowledge and experience. In many facilities, the facility manager or operations manager assumes all responsibility for emergency response activities.

The key objective in assigning overall responsibility is to ensure that corporate authority is in fact commensurate with that responsibility—a requirement that is more and more reflected in the consolidation of emergency response management duties within a corporate executive level function. For purposes of this text, the person having overall responsibility (and full authority) for the development and implementation of an emergency response program is referred to as the *emergency response manager* (ERM).

DEVELOPMENT OF EMERGENCY RESPONSE PLAN

Regardless of relevant regulatory standards and other legal and economic factors that influence the development of an emergency response program, and regardless of whether the objective is to create a document to be called a "RCRA Contingency Plan," "Spill Prevention Plan," "Emergency Response Plan," or "Emergency Action Plan," the development of a practical and effective emergency response program is essentially a *normative process*—a process whereby diverse technical information, social concerns, and health and safety objectives must be integrated and directed toward the practical implementation of strategies designed to achieve control of potential and actual emergencies.

As shown in Figure 13.1, the normative process involved in formulating a comprehensive emergency response plan may be viewed as consisting of three phases having distinct objectives:

1. Risk assessment phase: identification of the potential sources or cause of emergencies and the types and degrees of risk to be experienced by the work force and the public at large as well as corporate and local emergency response personnel
2. Safety judgment phase: establishment of levels of protection to be provided to persons at risk during an emergency
3. Making-safe strategy phase: formulation of specific procedures for achieving decided levels of protection

Risk Assessment Phase

The risk assessment phase (sometimes called simply "hazard assessment") is highly influenced by the concerns and considerations broadly attendant to the Bhopal (India) tragedy in which 4000 people died and 30,000–40,000 persons were seriously injured due to a leak of toxic gas at a Union Carbide pesticide plant—an event that, in the United States, became a prime motivation for the development of the Chemical Process Safety Regulations (29 CFR 1910.119). Even where these regulations do not specifically apply, they provide an excellent overview of the broad scope of modern emergency planning and are thereby highly instructive for any emergency response manager.

Various analytical techniques are germane to this phase—each of them providing different means for identifying potential sources of workplace emergencies and persons potentially at risk. Standard techniques include (a) preliminary hazard analysis, (b) what-if analysis, (c) hazard and operability analysis, (d) failure modes and effects analysis, (e) fault and event tree analysis, and (f) human reliability analysis.

Preliminary Hazard Analysis (PHA)

This technique focuses on the hazardous materials and major processing areas of a plant in order to identify hazards and potential accident

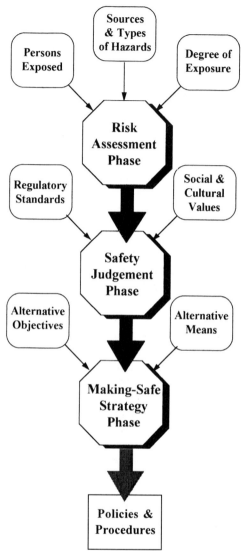

FIGURE 13.1   Key inputs to the three phases decision-making required for devising effective emergency response policies and procedures.

situations. It requires consideration of plant equipment, the interface among plant components, the operational environment, specific plant operations, and the physical layout of the plant. The objective of this technique is to assign a criticality ranking to each hazardous situation that may be envisioned, even in the absence of specific information about actual plant design features or operational procedures. It is particularly useful for identifying broadly defined causal chains (e.g., fire in materials processing can lead to explosion and release of toxic vapors; release of toxic vapors will be to the ambient atmosphere, and may threaten homes abutting company property; and so on) that can then be subjected to more detailed analysis.

What-If Analysis

In this analysis, experienced personnel formulate a series of questions that must be evaluated with respect to potential hazards identified in the preliminary hazard analysis. Typical questions might be of the type, "What if pump 23-b shuts off?" and "What if the operator forgets to empty the overflow tank at the end of the week?"

The basic strength of this approach is to define more precisely those causal chains that can lead to an emergency. In using this approach, the assessment team should explicitly consider two additional questions that are implicit in the question "What if?": "So what?" and "Says who?" For example, *what if* a chemical vapor escapes to the ambient atmosphere. The immediate effect is an atmospheric increase in the concentration of a particular chemical. The *so what* aspect of such an event depends on a host of considerations, such as the relative toxicity of the chemical, its capacity to cause irritation to living tissue, prevailing wind patterns that may disperse the vapor, the actual concentration of the vapor, and populations at potential risk. The result of a persistent posing of the question "So what?" is a chain or network of interrelated causes, effects, and circumstances. As the chain or network expands, the assessment team begins to understand the broad ramifications of a particular incident and becomes more adept at isolating particular factors or circumstances that can mean the difference between a minor and a major incident.

Each answer to the question "So what?" should be immediately addressed by the question "Says who?", which is a simple means of verifying the likelihood or plausibility of identified causal chains. Such verification may be on the basis of personal experience, professional opinion, or documented data and information. In many instances, answering the question "Says who" adequately will prove difficult, but it is nonetheless important because it forces attention on the need to test the veracity and relevance of information used to set policy.

Hazard and Operability Analysis (HAZOP)

This technique depends upon detailed information on the design and operation of the facility. In using this technique, the assessment team uses a standard set of *guide words* that, when combined with specific *process parameters*, lead to *resultant deviations* that may result in an emergency health and safety situation.

For example, the guide word "less" might be combined with the process parameter "pressure" to produce the resultant deviation "low pressure." The assessment team may then focus on the possible causes of "low pressure" (e.g., in a reactor) and the possible consequences of that "low pressure" (e.g., change in the rate of chemical reaction in the reactor).

Failure Modes and Effects Analysis

Closely related to "what if analysis," this technique focuses on the various failure modes of specific equipment and the effects of such failures on plant operations and human health and safety. Examples of questions that reflect this type of analysis when applied, say, to a control valve in a reactor vessel might include: What are the possible consequences of the control valve failing in the open position? In the closed position? What are the possible consequences if the control valve leaks while in the open or closed position?

Fault Tree and Event Tree Analysis

In fault tree analysis (FTA), a specific accident or plant failure (e.g., release of a toxic gas) is defined and all design, procedural and human errors leading to that event (called the "top event") are graphically modeled in a *fault tree*. The fault tree allows the analyst to define and rank particular groupings of external factors, equipment failures, and human errors (which are called "minimal cut sets") that are sufficient to lead to the top event.

While FTA focuses on failures in equipment or personnel that lead to the top event, event tree analysis (ETA) focuses on how successes or failures of specific in-place safety equipment, devices, and procedures may contribute to a developing emergency. This type of analysis is typically used to analyze very complex processes that incorporate several layers of safety systems or emergency procedures.

Human Reliability Analysis (HRA)

Generally conducted in parallel with other techniques, which tend to be equipment-oriented, this type of assessment focuses on factors that influence the actual job performance of personnel. In such an assessment, detailed descriptions of task requirements, the skills, knowledge and capabilities necessary for meeting each requirement, and error-prone situations that may develop during task performance are combined to isolate specific factors that, if ignored, might result in an emergency.

It is important that considered factors not be limited to those that are directly related to workplace conditions (e.g., ambient noise levels, which might affect a worker's concentration; work schedules, which can result in inattention due to fatigue), but are inclusive of the universe of factors that may influence workplace performance (e.g., personal financial difficulties, marital problems, substance abuse).

Regardless of the individual technique (or combination of techniques) employed, the ERM must ensure that the risk assessment process consider potential sources of emergency that derive from other than plant operations, including storms and floods, areawide fires and chemical releases, and terrorist acts. With regard to the latter, it is advisable that the ERM give particular attention to the fact that a perceived emergency may well be a "blind" to another.

For example, a telephoned bomb threat is likely to result in a plant evacuation within a matter of minutes, followed closely by the arrival of fire, police, and/or other specialized investigatory and emergency response units. In preparation for such an event, it is likely that the ERM and other members of the corporate emergency response team will have practiced plant evacuation, conducting the exercise just as it would in the case of any plant fire or toxic chemical release. However, in the case of a bomb threat, it may be the evacuating personnel or the emergency response personnel who are the real target of the threat and not the physical facility. Given this possibility, the prudent ERM would have ensured the implementation of appropriate procedures for detecting explosive or toxic charges that may be planted in evacuation assembly areas or precisely where emergency vehicles are likely to enter the premises.

Safety Judgment Phase

Having identified potential sources of emergencies as well as contributing factors and populations at risk, emergency planners must establish criteria regarding appropriate levels of protection for each at-risk population. This is a very difficult task precisely because it requires that judgments be made directly affecting the safety of human beings, therefore subject to seemingly endless ethical, moral, legal, and religious debate. The fact remains that there can be no such thing as a "100% guaranteed protection for all" in any real world situation, especially an emergency situation. The mere act of evacuating a group of people from a building puts some of those people at greater risk of suffering a heart attack or a fall injury than others; panic can kill as effectively as fire. Of course, individual physical and psychological conditions that ensure some differential distribution of risks regardless of any effort to the contrary are not excuses for inaction. In fact, it is precisely the recognition of a differential distribution of risks that becomes the basis of an effective emergency response plan.

In the United States, regulatory guidance (OSHA and EPA) regarding the level of protection for personnel having specific responsibility in an emergency involving hazardous chemicals is based on the following typology of emergency responders, which includes members of so-called HAZMAT (for "hazardous materials") teams. The designation "HAZMAT" always denotes personnel who are expected to perform work in close proximity to a hazardous substance while handling or controlling actual or potential leaks or spills, and should not be confused with other emergency personnel, such as members of a fire brigade.

- Level 1: responders who are most likely to witness or discover a hazardous substance release and to initiate an emergency response sequence by notifying the proper authorities
- Level 2: police, firefighters, and rescue personnel who are part of the initial response to a release or potential release of hazardous substances
- Level 3: HAZMAT technicians, who are the first level specifically charged with trying to contain a release of hazardous substances
- Level 4: HAZMAT specialists, who respond with and provide support to HAZMAT technicians and have more specific knowledge of hazardous substances
- Level 5: on-scene "incident commanders" or "senior officials in charge," who assume control of the emergency response incident scene and coordinate all activities and communications

The various levels of responders indicated above can be cross-referenced with various levels of *protective ensembles* (Table 13.1) to meet regulatory requirements regarding personal protective clothing and equipment, such as the requirements of 29 CFR 1910.120. While the above typology of responders gives heavy emphasis to protection from hazardous chemicals, other types of emergency situations and job requirements require other regulatory inputs to the planning process, such as 29 CFR 1910.156 standards that specifically apply to members of a fire brigade.

In the process of coordinating with community-based emergency responders, including local fire departments, the ERM must give special attention to the adequacy of protective clothing and equipment available to external responders with respect to the specific hazards associated with company operations. This is often a critical concern because the local firefighter or other local responder, who is usually the first responder to an emergency, typically does not have direct access to the kind of personnel protection devices that are standard equipment for a formal HAZMAT team, which can often arrive on-site only well after an emergency has progressed.

In many cases, for example, local firefighters will not be equipped with chemically impervious protective clothing that would be required to retrieve personnel trapped within a company facility where highly toxic chemicals are used or stored. In some situations, companies have purchased such clothing and maintain it for use by local firefighters. Sometimes a company may also supply the local fire department with additional materials and specialized equipment, including antidotes to toxic chemicals used on site, specialized monitoring devices, and materials that firefighters can use to disinfect clothing and equipment contaminated by especially dangerous chemicals.

Having determined the level of protection appropriate to both in-plant and external emergency responders, the ERM must consider the degree of protection that may be appropriate for persons who might otherwise become exposed to hazards as the result of an emergency, including company personnel not directly involved as emergency responders and the general public. The approach here is most practicably one of providing for (a) emergency first aid and transportation to appropriate medical facilities, (b) contractor services that may be immediately required to achieve containment of the emergency, and (c) specialized services regarding the evaluation of key factors that can determine the extent and magnitude of a developing emergency, such as computer-assisted projections of the dynamics of air and water plumes of contaminated materials. While such activities and services become of central importance during the third phase of program development, which involves the formulation of specific policies and procedures, it is important to consider them in this phase so that minimal objectives and requirements can be specified early in the development process. Some examples of judgments to be made in this phase regarding each of the above types of services are as follows:

1. First aid services:

    - What must the company provide in terms of personnel training and first aid materials and supplies?
    - What types of temporary shelters may be required to administer first aid under inclement weather conditions or to protect both first aid responders and injured persons from further contamination?
    - How are persons to be identified as being in need of first aid, and what type of communication requirements must be met to ensure that persons in need have immediate access to first aid services?

2. Contractor services:

TABLE 13.1 Types of Protective Ensembles[a]

a

Level of Protection and Equipment	Overview of Protection	Conditions for Use and Limitations

A
 	
Recommended:
• Pressure-demand, full-facepiece SCBA or pressure-demand supplied air respirator with escape SCBA
• Fully encapsulating, chemical resistant suit
• Inner chemical-resistant gloves
• Chemical resistant safety boots/shoes
• Two-way radio
 	
Optional:
• Cooling unit
• Coveralls
• Long cotton underwear
• Hard hat
• Disposable gloves and boot covers
	The highest available level of respiratory, skin, and eye protection	• The chemical substance has been identified and requires the highest level of protection for skin, eyes, and the respiratory system based on either:
		
		  1. measured (or potential for) high concentration of atmospheric vapors, gases, or particulates, or
		  2. site operations and work functions involving a high potential for splash, immersion, or exposure to unexpected vapors, gases, or particulates of materials that are harmful to skin or capable of being absorbed through the intact skin.
		
		• Substances with a high degree of hazard to the skin are known or suspected to be present, and skin contact is possible.
		• Operations must be conducted in confined, poorly ventilated areas until the absence of conditions requiring Level A protection is determined.
		• Fully encapsulating suit materials must be compatible with the substances involved.

B
 	
Recommended:
• Pressure-demand, full facepiece SCBA or pressure-demand supplied air respirator with escape SCBA
• Chemical-resistant clothing
• Inner and outer chemical-resistant gloves
• Chemical resistant safety boots/shoes
• Hard Hat
• Two-way Radio
 	
Optional:
• Coveralls
• Disposable boot covers
• Face shield
• Long cotton underwear
	The same level of respiratory protection but less skin protection than Level A.
	
	This the minimum level recommended for initial site entries until the hazards have been further identified.
		• The type and atmospheric concentration of substances have been identified and require a high level of respiratory protection, but less skin protection. This involves atmospheres
		
		  -- with IDLH concentrations of specific substances that do not represent a severe skin hazard, or
		
		  -- that do not meet the criteria for use of air-purifying respirators.
		
		• Atmosphere contains less than 19.5 % oxygen.
		• Presence of incompletely identified vapors or gases is indicated by direct-reading organic vapor detection instrument, but vapors and gases are not suspected of containing high levels of chemicals harmful to skin or capable of being absorbed through intact skin.
		• Use only when highly unlikely that the work will generate either high concentrations of vapors, gases, or particulates or splashes of material will affect exposed skin.

continues

continued

b

Level of Protection and Equipment	Overview of Protection	Conditions for Use and Limitations
C **Recommended:** • Full-facepiece, air purifying, canister equipped respirator • Chemical resistant clothing • Inner and outer chemical resistant gloves • Chemical resistant safety boots/shoes • Hard hat • Two-way radio **Optional:** • Coveralls • Disposable boot covers • Face shield • Escape mask • Long cotton underwear	The same level of skin protection as Lervel B, but a lower level of respiratory protection	• Atmospheric contaminants, liquid splashes, or other direct contact will not adversely affect any exposed skin. • The types of air contaminants have been identified, concentrations measured, and a canister is available that can remove the contaminant. • All criteria for the use of air-purifying respirators are met. • Atmospheric concentration of chemicals must not exceed IDLH levels. • The atmosphere must contain at least 19.5 % oxygen.
D **Recommended:** • Coveralls • Safety boots/shoes • Safety glasses or chemical splash goggles • Hard hat **Optional:** • Gloves • Escape mask • Face shield	No respiratory protection; minimal skin protection	• The atmosphere contains no known hazard. • Work functions preclude splashes, immersion, or the potential for unexpected inhalation of or contact with hazardous levels of any chemicals. • This level should not be worn in the Exclusion Zone. • The atmosphere must contain at least 19.5 % oxygen.

[a] Adapted from materials provided by NIOSH, OSHA, U.S. Coast Guard, and U.S. EPA.

• Do local contractors have direct 24-hr access to appropriate equipment (e.g., trucks, front end loaders) and supplies (e.g., sand, soil) to accomplish containment objectives?
• What protective equipment or clothing will be required by equipment operators or other contractor laborers?

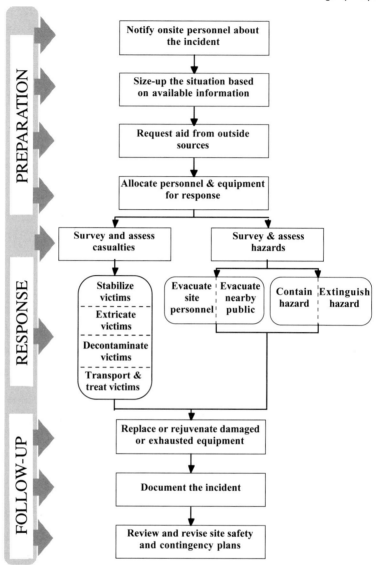

FIGURE 13.2 Basic emergency response operations *(adapted from materials provided by NIOSH, OSHA, U.S. Coast Guard, and U.S. EPA).*

3. Other specialized services:

- What is the 24-hr availability of computer hardware and software as well as of trained personnel that may be needed to project the direction, rate of travel and concentration of chemical contaminants?

- What on-site data and information are necessary as inputs to computerized atmospheric or hydrologic models?

Making-Safe Strategy Phase

In this phase, the objective is to assess and select from among alternative means for achieving the standards and objectives previously identified and, finally, to develop specific policies and procedures that govern all aspects of emergency response. As shown in Figure 13.2, policies and procedures should address three basic types of emergency response activities: (a) preparation activities, which are undertaken immediately upon discovery of a potential or actual emergency and prior to the initiation of any response, (b) response activities, which include all efforts to control the emergency and provide assistance to affected persons, and (c) follow-up activities, which focus on postemergency actions to bring the company back to a state of emergency readiness, including revisions to emergency plans necessitated by the experience of the now-past emergency. It must here be emphasized that the usual tendency is for companies to concentrate on the response to an emergency at the expense of attention given to both preparatory or follow-up actions—which is an extremely dangerous approach to emergency planning. Effective emergency planning always requires equally serious attention to all three types of actions.

The ultimate key to any emergency response is communication—among in-plant personnel and with external emergency response resources—and it is precisely communication that is so often subject to serious error and oversight because it depends upon so many interdependent needs and conditions, including:

- the necessity of establishing clear and concise criteria that in-plant personnel can use to recognize that a potential or actual emergency exists
- the proclivity of production-oriented managers and other personnel to ignore potentially dangerous situations or to assume that such situations are "part of the job" or that they are the responsibility of somebody else
- the need for a clear line of in-plant and external communication that is operable over a 24-hr period and under all conceivable conditions, including power outages
- the need for a standardized format for and substantive content of information to be communicated

- the lack of any clear understanding of chains of command, among in-plant personnel, and especially between in-plant authorities and external emergency responders

While various regulations stipulate that the ERM must be on-site within a reasonable period of time (e.g., 15–20 min) after the first notification of an emergency, the ERM is well advised that even such an apparently short interval of time can, in fact, be an eternity in an actual emergency. An on-site person should always be delegated the full authority of the ERM until such a time that the ERM arrives on site and takes control.

However well conceived and implemented, policies and procedures regarding in-plant and external communication are, of course, essentially to no avail in the absence of precise policies and procedures governing response and follow-up actions. There can be no doubt that, even for small companies, the collection of policies and procedures that document a comprehensive approach to the management of emergencies can be (and most often is) an extensive compendium that represents a significant investment in time and effort—time and effort that is too often wasted because so little time is spent ensuring that personnel can implement those policies and procedures efficiently and effectively.

REFINEMENT OF EMERGENCY RESPONSE PLAN

Once initial policies and procedures have been developed, they should be subjected to a series of exercises designed to test and refine them. Such exercises are of three basic types: (a) in-plant testing, (b) table-top exercise, and (c) field exercise.

In-plant testing involves a variety of "walk-through" exercises, including practice evacuations, mock drills for in-plant responders, and round-table workshops that focus on a particular type of emergency situation, such as a leak in a chemical reactor. These exercises may be conducted at different levels of readiness, starting with preannounced and extending to unannounced exercises. However, in each case, exercises are restricted to in-house personnel and, though involving training (through practice), are finally geared to testing the adequacy of proposed policies and procedures and to fine-tune them.

A table-top exercise is essentially a staged mock-up of an emergency that is presented in such a way as to elicit the responses of the emergency team under simulated conditions. While it can be conducted solely by in-house personnel, it is ideally conducted by both in-plant and external emergency responders.

In its typical format, a table-top exercise is a scenario of an emergency; the details are given to the team of in-plant and external responders in piecemeal fashion, beginning first with notification of the emergency situation. Over a period of several hours, details that reflect the ongoing development of the emergency and the consequences of decisions made by the team are added. Maps, scale models of the plant, and other informational aids, including staged telephone calls, news reports, and computer readouts are used to provide as much a sense of reality as possible. Upon completion of the emergency scenario, a detailed debriefing of the team is conducted to evaluate the performance of the team and devise alternative strategies for improving performance.

On the basis of in-plant testing and table-top exercises, field exercises may be designed both to test procedures and to train personnel under the actual constraints of weather, plant layout, transportation routes, and the availability of external responders. As with any exercise, a field enactment of an emergency may simulate different degrees of reality; the response team must imagine certain conditions and deal with role-playing "victims" and simulated smoke or spills of "prop" chemicals.

Whatever the exercise, the ERM should clearly understand that in-plant testing and table-top and field exercises are not only effective means for refining policies and procedures for managing emergencies, but also for training personnel. Table-top and field exercises are also especially valuable for acquainting external emergency responders with actual plant operations and layout—information that, in a real emergency, can be vital not only with regard to their own safety, but to the safety of plant personnel and the surrounding community.

SITE SAFETY PLAN

Because the emergency response plan is basically a compilation of all policies and procedures regarding potential and actual emergencies, and because such a plan—if properly developed—is typically a relatively large compendium, it is advisable that a company use that plan to develop, where possible, generic plans that focus on particular types of emergencies. One example is a site safety plan.

A site safety plan may focus, for example, on those particular aspects of the company's emergency response plan that pertain to an on-site chemical spill or, even more specifically, to a chemical spill not involving the hazard of fire or explosion. Another site safety plan may focus on decontamination during and after an emergency involving exposure to hazardous chemicals.

Such plans are commonly developed in the United States by governmental agencies, such as the U.S. Coast Guard or the U.S. Department of Transportation, which have the responsibility of responding to specific types of emergencies. They are also useful in companies that, regardless of size, present a variety of distinctly different hazards. For companies that fall within the purview of 29 CFR 1910.120, a site safety plan is required by regulations.

The primary advantage of a generic site safety plan is that it can be presented in a much abridged format as compared to a comprehensive emergency response plan. In many instances, the format may approach that of a checklist that requires the in-plant responder to take clearly defined steps in a precise sequence. While the contents of a site safety plan will vary depending upon the purpose of the plan and any relevant regulatory requirements, basic information and procedures may be organized under the following types of headings:

- description of the type of emergency and minimum information required
- in-plant and external notification requirements
- on-site responsible personnel
- criteria to be applied in evaluating levels of emergency
- evacuation requirements
- personnel protective clothing and equipment required (by task)
- personnel monitoring requirements
- communication procedures
- site control procedures (entry and access to defined zones; decontamination)
- emergency medical care
- postemergency actions and documentation

SITE CONTROL

The control of access to plant facilities and areas is a vital aspect of any health and safety program, in both routine and emergency situations. Under routine conditions, site control is the basic means of minimizing the exposure of personnel to hazardous circumstances and the potential for vandalism or terrorist acts. During an emergency, site control is essential to control the exposure of responding personnel and to ensure that the work of both in-plant and external emergency responders can be conducted in an unimpeded fashion.

In considering the practical advantages and disadvantages involved in implementing routine site control policies, many companies tend to quickly perceive site control as too inconvenient, too costly, and too complex—arguments that may or may not have some validity but which are most often simply convenient rationalizations for maintaining a policy of casual access that is based on historical practice and not on any other consideration. In such instances, it is likely that site control will be seriously evaluated as a basic element of the corporate health and safety program only after an actual emergency is traced to the wrong person being in the wrong place and doing the wrong thing—an occurrence that, regrettably, is increasingly commonplace not only as a result of purposeful terrorist acts but also the vandalism of disgruntled employees, acts of revenge by terminated employees, and the otherwise innocent actions of plant visitors, contractors, and other personnel who do not understand either the risks presented by company operations or the potential consequences of their seemingly harmless actions. The old excuse "I didn't know the gun was loaded" is today an outdated bromide and cannot be tolerated in any responsible program of workplace health and safety.

In the workplace, there are many guns and they are always loaded. Routine site control begins with detailed knowledge of "where the guns are" and "how they can be fired" and concerns itself with restricting access to them on the basis of defined job requirements. Essential elements in an effective site control program for routine operations therefore minimally consist of:

1. An overview map of the plant, showing property lines, routes of access, major structures, and locations of sensitive operations— i.e., those that are of particular concern as potential sources of an emergency (electrical transformer vault, chemical reactor vessels) or as particularly hazardous to emergency responders (e.g., a hazardous waste storage area, storage tanks for hazardous chemical feedstock)
2. Floor plans for individual buildings or facilities, showing precise location of hazardous operations or materials
3. Written job descriptions, including summaries of required personnel access to plant facilities and operations
4. Summary descriptions and locations of areas and operations having restricted access by in-plant personnel and other persons (e.g., visitors, vendors, contractors, consultants, service personnel), including in-place signs and other warnings of restricted access, restrictions imposed by job category, time and type of activity, and restrictions regarding personal protective clothing and equipment
5. Procedures and devices used to enforce restrictions and to document compliance and oversight

With respect to site control in an actual emergency situation, the ERM must meet the requirements of regulations (e.g., 29 CFR 1910.120) that may be relevant to the designated duties of in-plant emergency responders and must also be aware of the requirements imposed by external emergency responders, such as the fire department or a local HAZMAT team. In emergencies requiring the use of external responders, the ERM is strongly advised to act in all ways to facilitate the implementation of site control procedures imposed by external authorities. Under no circumstance should any company policy or procedure be used to contravene the emergency response procedures of the fire department, local HAZMAT team, or any other local authority required to provide emergency assistance.

EMERGENCY DATA AND INFORMATION

Second only to the responsibility of the company to implement plant evacuation in the event of an actual emergency is the company's responsibility to provide external responders with the data and information they need to implement their response and to protect their own personnel.

Increasingly, companies use standardized *lockout boxes* to provide the local fire department 24-hr access not only to a facility master key (which has long been common) but also to basic data and information, including (a) overview maps and diagrams of company property, access points, emergency equipment, and site-specific hazards, (b) detailed floor plans, and (c) inventory and location of hazardous chemicals. Of course, the fire department also has access to information about a company through Section 302 of SARA.

The first information required by a fire chief arriving on scene is whether or not all persons have been evacuated from the affected area—information that cannot be provided by the ERM except through active communication with in-plant personnel who have specific responsibility for monitoring the evacuation process and reporting (via radio) from assembly areas to the ERM.

Unless directed otherwise by the fire chief or the coordinator of the HAZMAT team, the ERM should remain immediately available to provide whatever additional information or assistance may be necessary. To meet this objective, the ERM should maintain direct contact with key personnel who may best be able to provide that information or assistance, such as the plant engineer, the hazardous waste coordinator, or the chemical hygiene officer—persons who, of course, should already have been identified in the progress of developing the corporate emergency response plan and who have participated in the relevant in-plant testing and table-top and field exercises.

Of crucial importance is the management of persons who have been evacuated. Inclement weather, potential exposure to smoke and other fumes produced by a fire, as well as other considerations, such as potential interference of evacuees with movement of emergency equipment and notification of family members, may require the ERM to move evacuees to shelter or otherwise provide for their safety or comfort. However, the ERM should take no action in this or any other regard without first coordinating with the responsible fire or HAZMAT official.

Finally, no discussion of the various responsibilities regarding the communication of data and information about an ongoing emergency is complete without giving emphasis to the necessity to manage information provided to the mass media. The potential physical interference of media personnel with the orderly progress of emergency response efforts (e.g., news helicopters landing in an active emergency response zone), as well as the indirect effect of broadcast news promoting the convergence of "gawkers" and "thrill seekers" to emergency sites is well documented throughout the world. In the modern world, managing the public relations aspects of an emergency becomes intertwined with managing the actual emergency response effort and cannot be disregarded.

CHAPTER 14

MANAGEMENT OF CHANGE

BACKGROUND

In 1992, the U.S. OSHA implemented its final rule that is most often referred to as the "Chemical Process Safety Regulation," which is a much abridged name from the more formal appellation, "Process Safety Management of Highly Hazardous Chemicals, Explosives and Blasting Agents." The final rule actually consists of two major sets of regulations: one dealing with the management of explosive and blasting agents (29 CFR 1910.109); the other, with the management of "highly hazardous chemicals" (29 CFR 1910.119). Section (l) of 29 CFR 1910.119 defines the objective of "Management of Change."

Those companies that handle any of more than 135 listed chemicals at or above so-called "threshold quantities" (pounds of chemical) must comply with the provisions of 29 CFR 1910.119. However, even a company that does not fall within the regulatory purview of the process safety regulations is well advised to consider the development of a management of change program.

The basic objective of any management of change program is to ensure that good engineering principles and practices are always used when designing, constructing, operating, and maintaining facilities. This objective requires the recognition that even relatively small and seemingly innocuous changes associated with facility design, construction, operations, and maintenance may actually result in unacceptable health and safety hazards. It is worthwhile to review a few examples of the kinds of changes that prompt concern for the management of change in industry.

Example 14.1 In a chemical processing plant, a pressure-release valve on a chemical reactor is vented by a stainless steel pipe that runs horizontally from the reactor through an external wall. Over time, it is noticed that water condensate from the pipe runs down the exterior wall, leaving a stain. The maintenance department, having determined that the stain is a minor aesthetic problem that can be easily rectified, attaches a 15-foot section of vertical pipe to the horizontal vent pipe, which allows the condensate to be released immediately above ground. However, in the subsequent winter during an extended period of severe cold, the condensate, now draining through the narrow bore vertical pipe, freezes and forms an ice plug that extends through much of the pipe and thereby occludes the release of pressure. The end result is an explosion of the reactor vessel, with the release of highly toxic and corrosive chemical reagents.

Example 14.2   As part of a comprehensive fire prevention and control plan, a company implements a new alarm system that is electronically coupled to the exhaust drive motors, shutting off several laboratory hoods used for the handling and processing of particularly hazardous chemicals in an R&D laboratory. This practice, which ensures that hood exhaust cannot exacerbate the spread of a fire, is standard practice and is typically recommended by corporate insurance companies and fire departments. Also in conformity with good fire prevention and control practice, the company implements regularly scheduled tests of the alarm system, which are immediately preceded by an announcement over the plant public address system that a test of the fire alarm is imminent and that personnel should continue with routine operations. However, during one particular test, routine laboratory operations included the use of particularly volatile and toxic chemicals which, because of the automatic shutdown of hood motors, escaped into the laboratory and adjoining facilities. Not only had the facility manager responsible for initiating the alarm test failed to coordinate with the laboratory manager regarding ongoing laboratory operations, but the manager had to learn "the hard way" that the company did not have any in-plant means for immediately overriding the electronic linkage of the fire alarm and hood motors, with the result that a large number of personnel were exposed to dangerous levels of toxic chemicals.

Example 14.3   In its effort to achieve a significant improvement in corporate health care, a company establishes an in-plant emergency medical department which is staffed by a registered nurse for each of three shifts. The nurses work under the supervision of a consulting licensed physician who is available for consultation but who is not on-site. During the third shift, which is primarily devoted to the charging of chemical reactor vessels and other materials-handling and processing equipment, a chemical hopper located on the second floor of the facility malfunctions, with the subsequent spillage of dry chemical feedstock to the first floor dispensing area, which partially engulfs one person who is nonetheless able to extricate himself without any physical injury. Upon arriving on scene, the nurse uses water and a sponge to remove most of the chemical powder from the worker's hair, face, neck and hands and directs him to shower. The nurse does not know that the chemical, essentially nontoxic in dry form, is highly toxic once solubilized, primarily because of its rapid absorption through the skin directly into the blood. The otherwise uninjured worker dies of chemical poisoning within 20 min of receiving initial treatment.

In each of these examples, it is quite easy to exercise the proverbial wisdom of hindsight to assign blame to individuals—to the maintenance supervisor who should have known that the water condensate would freeze; to the facility manager who should have known that hood shutdown would result in the fugitive fumes; and to the nurse who should have known that the solubilized toxic chemical would be rapidly absorbed through skin. However, of course, assigning individual blame retroactively does not absolve a company of corporate responsibility for acting proactively to ensure health and safety—and the basic tenet of any proactive effort is to assume that humans most often exercise much less than perfect judgment.

In each of these cases, the sequence of events that ultimately resulted in significant health and safety risks began with some type of change—a change in facility design, a change in equipment, and a change in procedure. Management of change simply reflects corporate recognition that any type of change, even one specifically implemented to improve health and safety, always involves unknown or unimagined or simply overlooked factors and circumstances that can result in tragedy—and that, over and above the personal responsibilities of persons who implement the change, the company itself has broad responsibility for ensuring that the possible ramifications of proposed changes are properly assessed in a proactive manner.

TYPOLOGY OF CHANGE

The practical implementation of a management of change (MOC) program requires clear criteria for distinguishing between those changes in plant operations, design and features that have no reasonable likelihood of resulting in a threat to health and safety and those that do.

Under 29 CFR 1910.119, specific exemption from MOC requirements is granted any change that is a *replacement in kind*, which is any replacement of a part (i.e., equipment, machinery, or material) or procedure that satisfies ongoing design specifications that pertain to the performance or role of that part or procedure in plant processes involving regulated chemicals. Within the limited context of this regulatory authority, MOC procedures must address the following issues with regard to any change that is not a replacement in kind:

- the technical basis for the proposed change
- the impact of the change on safety and health
- modification of operating procedures appropriate to the change and its related risks
- the time period required for preparing and implementing the change
- authorization requirements attendant to the change

The usual means for addressing these issues is the integration of MOC procedures with existing in-plant approval and authorization procedures, especially standard internal work request and work order procedures. This approach is eminently practical whether a company falls within the jurisdictional purview of 29 CFR 1910.119 or, if not subject to these regulations, simply chooses to implement an MOC policy as one component of a comprehensive health and safety program, an option that is increasingly exercised by companies in the United States and elsewhere. In fact, MOC is widely recognized as a state-of-the-art business management practice regardless of legal authority.

Where MOC is practiced routinely and regardless of regulatory jurisdiction, corporate decision-making procedures involving work requests and work orders provide specific lines of authority and responsibility for all potential changes, including those involving replacement in kind (most often called *change in kind*) as well as *changes not in kind*—in fact, the typology of changes, inclusive of some range of changes from negligible to severe risk to health and safety, is precisely reflected by the increased level of authority required to implement the change.

For example, Figure 14.1 is an overview of an MOC procedure that provides for three basic types of changes, each type being defined essentially by the level of authority required to implement it:

- Level 1: a change that may be authorized solely by the department supervisor who, on the basis of written criteria provided by the company, determines that the change is a "change in kind" and thereby presents negligible hazard or risk.
- Level 2: a change that does not meet the criteria for a Level 1 change and which, with the concurrence of the corporate safety officer, may be implemented by the department manager only after completion of a "management record of change," which is essentially a checklist that directs the manager's assessment of the change and its implementation; in this case, a Level 2 change is known to present more than a negligible health and safety risk, but one that is relatively uncomplicated and easily controlled.
- Level 3: a change that does not meet the criteria for a Level 1 change and that, by its nature or complexity, is judged to require the attention of the highest corporate authority, including the safety officer, the safety

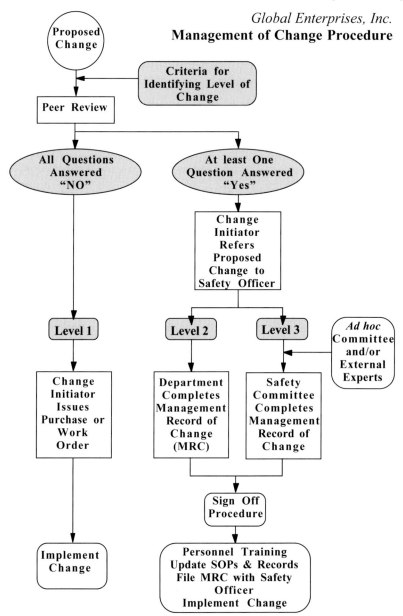

FIGURE 14.1 Example of flow diagram of decision-making requirements for the management of change in a manufacturing plant. Shaded areas are items that must be cross-referenced to informational requirements as specified in other corporate documents (see Figures 14.2 and 14.3).

committee, the facility manager and other selected corporate personnel, and, possibly, external consultants and experts.

The procedure depicted in Figure 14.1 clearly requires an assessment of the hazards and risks associated with even a change in kind that typically meets the criterion for a replacement in kind, which is exempted from MOC requirements under 29 CFR 1910.119. This procedure also allows MOC to be exercised for all changes, as opposed to just those changes that are pertinent to chemical processes falling within regulatory purview. Because this procedure goes beyond the regulatory constraint of 29 CFR 1910.119 and is therefore more inclusive of MOC in general industry, and because it requires the integrated efforts of personnel at various levels of corporate management (e.g., departmental supervisors and managers, safety officer, and corporate executives), it is worth expanding upon both the strengths and the limitations of this particular procedure, which is henceforth referred to as the "integrated MOC procedure."

DISTRIBUTION OF RESPONSIBILITY AND AUTHORITY

The underlying assumption of the integrated MOC procedure shown in Figure 14.1 is that both the responsibility and the authority regarding workplace health and safety is appropriately distributed throughout the company, from departmental supervisors and managers to the highest level of executives. Such a pervasive involvement of corporate structure and management with health and safety is, regrettably, in direct opposition to the more frequent practice of investing a particular person (e.g., the safety or the regulatory compliance officer) with sole responsibility (though not often with commensurate authority). There are several good reasons that this latter practice, however, is fast becoming an historical artifact, especially with regard to the management of change:

1. The number, scope, and complexity of modern regulations regarding workplace health and safety are themselves sufficient to tax even the most ardent efforts of a corporate safety officer, but they do not define the limits of responsibility, which are also directly influenced by broad environmental regulations that increasingly require health and safety assessment and management, by nonregulatory but nonetheless legal considerations, including corporate and personal financial and criminal responsibility, and, last but not least, by the demands and obligations of personal and social ethics and morals.

2. Despite the best efforts of a safety officer to develop and integrate highly diverse health and safety policies, success and failure are ultimately measured in terms of what actually happens in the workplace on a day-to-

day basis—and what actually happens does not automatically follow from the dictates of health and safety policies and programs. What actually happens depends largely on the vastly greater number of factors and conditions, including work schedules, facility operations and maintenance, personnel actions, and inventory management, that typically lie beyond the jurisdictional authority or technical competence of the safety officer.

3. Regardless of in-plant assignations of both responsibility and authority regarding environmental quality and human health and safety, there is broad legal, political, and social agreement that neither corporations nor corporate owners nor corporate executives can "contract away" or "trade off" or otherwise divest themselves of their own responsibility. In matters involving environmental quality and human health and safety, the key question is increasingly not "what *did* the company's key decision-makers know?" but, rather, "what *should* they have known?"—a question that contravenes any semblance of legitimacy imparted by those intricately devised job titles and levels of command that have historically camouflaged personal *irresponsibility* with official *nonresponsibility*.

Management of change procedures that do not recognize that the control of workplace hazards and risks require the integrated efforts, experience, and knowledge of persons having diverse job responsibilities and that even a corporate safety officer must function more as the coordinator of plantwide contributions to health and safety objectives than the sole provider of health and safety advice and direction are bound to fail. On the other hand, if the responsibility and authority for the management of change is to be distributed among diverse personnel, it is absolutely necessary that clear and concise criteria are established for coordinating their individual efforts.

MANAGEMENT OF CHANGE CRITERIA

Where an integrated MOC procedure is implemented, criteria must be provided to departmental level personnel that can be used to (a) identify the various levels of change included in the MOC program, and (b) facilitate any disagreements among key personnel regarding the assessment of level. As a general rule, MOC criteria should be established only after categorical types of representative changes have been identified for each department, usually as the result of "brainstorming" sessions conducted in each department and in which departmental personnel at all levels review routine as well as emergency activities and in-plant accident records. After department review, departmental supervisors and managers throughout the plant should then convene to develop a master list of types of changes to be addressed by the MOC program. It is this master list that ultimately provides the basis for designing a change request form that provides direction for the implementation of MOC.

An example of a two-page MOC change request form is provided in Figures 14.2 and 14.3. In this example, the form must be completed by the person who is responsible for initiating a proposed change in a company where corporate policy declares that, for purposes of MOC, "a change includes any and all changes, including (but not limited to) procedures, practices, protocols, policies, schedules, equipment, supplies, materials, items, raw materials, personnel assignments, and training that are (or may be) directly or indirectly pertinent to the structure, design, operation and maintenance of the facility."

In this particular example, the initiator of the proposed change is typically the departmental supervisor who uses the first page of the MOC change request (Figure 14.2) to document the nature of the proposed change, a summary finding of the level of change (as defined in Figure 14.1), and department personnel that the initiator consulted in the process whereby the initiator actually determined the level of change. Note that this company also requires certification of the initiator's determination by a second person who is identified as specifically authorized to do so.

The second page of the MOC change request (Figure 14.3) contains 11 basic criteria to be considered by the initiator of the proposed change in determining level of change. In this example, the company has designed these criteria in the form of questions that can be answered "yes" or "no," with any single "yes" response being sufficient to require coordination with the safety officer and, possibly, with even higher corporate authority (Figure 14.1).

Several aspects of this type of approach should be given particular emphasis:

1. The first criterion included in Figure 14.3 pertains to the potential relationship between the proposed change and any of 15 written corporate programs related to environmental quality and worker health and safety. Because this change request form is completed at the departmental level, the assumption made by this particular company is clearly that departmental supervisors and managers are thoroughly familiar with the provisions of these written programs and understand the direct relevance of these programs to departmental activities. In the absence of a persistent training effort and of effective quality control mechanisms that ensure and enforce such departmental understanding and responsibility, the inclusion of such a criterion in a change request form is inappropriate.

2. All of the criteria presume that the initiator of any proposed change has sufficiently extensive experience in plant operations to ensure a

Global Enterprises, Inc.

| For Safety Officer's Use Only |
| Log Number |
| Process Code |

Management of Change
Request & Determination of Level

Name of Person Initiating Change

Description of Proposed Change

Individuals Consulted
Name   **Department**

I certify that I have consulted with the above individuals for the purpose of completing the reverse side of this form. On the basis of the information included on this form, I determine that the proposed change described above ...

☐ Is a Level 1 Change   ☐ Must be referred to the Global Safety Officer for his determination

_____   _____
Signature of Change Initiator   Date

I certify that I have reviewed this determination and hereby agree with the above determination.

_____   _____
Signature of Authorized Person   Date

Page 1 of 2

FIGURE 14.2 First page of a "management of change request and determination of level" form used by a manufacturing plant. This page describes the proposed change and provides basic documentation regarding the initiator of that change and other personnel consulted for the purpose of assessing the status of the proposed change in light of corporate policy (Figure 14.1).

Global Enterprises, Inc.

Managment of Change Request & Determination of Level

> The supervisor or manager of the department responsible for carrying out the proposed change must complete this form and submit the completed form to the Global Safety Officer

If the answer to each of the following questions is "no," the proposed change is a Level 1 change. If the answer to *any* question is "yes," the proposed change must be referred to the Global Safety Officer (or his designate).

Will the Proposed Change ...

	YES	NO
1. Require any modification of any of the following Global Programs:		
• Lockout/Tagout	☐	☐
• Confined Space Entry	☐	☐
• Hot Work Permit	☐	☐
• Respiratory Protection	☐	☐
• Bloodborne Pathogens	☐	☐
• Hazard Communication	☐	☐
• Laboratory Standard	☐	☐
• Electrical Safety	☐	☐
• Hazardous Waste Contingency Plan	☐	☐
• Hearing Conservation Program	☐	☐
• Process Safety Management	☐	☐
• Ergonomic Safety	☐	☐
• Good Manufacturing Processes	☐	☐
• Personal Protective Clothing & Equipment	☐	☐
• Stormwater Pollution Prevention	☐	☐
2. Require more than routine coordination with other departments	☐	☐
3. Result in any change in equipment or piping	☐	☐
4. Result in any change in structural design or physical layout	☐	☐
5. Result in any change in raw materials or by-products	☐	☐
6. Result in a significant change in energy consumption	☐	☐
7. Result in any interruption of automatic or manual signaling devices or alarms, automatic process controls, alarms or instrumentation	☐	☐
8. Interfere with the normal functioning of any safety or emergency equipment (e.g., sprinklers, ventilation, emergency lighting)	☐	☐
9. Significantly affect the routine on-site work of external contractors or consultants	☐	☐
10. Result in a significant change in operating procedures or process directions	☐	☐
11. Result in a change in process parameters (e.g., temperature, pressure) beyond documented operational limits	☐	☐

Page 2 of 2

FIGURE 14.3 Second page of the "management of change request and determination of level" form. This page must be completed by the initiator of the proposed change and is the basis for determining the "level" of change as required by corporate policy (Figure 14.1).

reasonable "comfort level" in making judgments. Inexperienced personnel are likely to defeat the attempt to distribute MOC responsibility through-out appropriate corporate levels by consistently determining the proposed change to be (in this example) a level 2 or level 3 change—i.e., one requiring action at a higher authority. Safety officers and other managers having over-all MOC responsibility should therefore periodically (e.g., at least annually) review MOC determinations conducted at the departmental level to evaluate the appropriateness of personnel assigned MOC responsibility.

3. The requirement that the initiation of the proposed change must consult with co-workers in the progress of determining the level of change is particularly important because it fosters the discussion and assessment of health and safety issues at the floor level of the company and thereby gives practical validation to the precept that "safety is everybody's responsibility."

Whatever the format used for MOC criteria, and regardless of the specific responsibilities of key personnel, it should be expected that disagree-ments as to the potential significance of proposed changes will occur. The MOC program must therefore provide clear means for resolving such conflicts.

For example, where an integrated MOC procedure requires that the primary determination of "change in kind" be made by a departmental su-pervisor (Figure 14.1), it is very possible that the departmental supervisor and the safety officer will disagree. In such a case, the conflict may most easily be resolved by the safety officer signing the "change request" form and thereby taking full responsibility for determining that the proposed change is a "change in kind" that requires no further action.

In many instances, it may be desirable to resolve conflict simply by opting for the more stringent assessment—as, for example, when a depart-mental manager and the safety officer may disagree as to a particular pro-posed change being either a level 2 or a level 3 type of change (Figure 14.1).

MANAGEMENT RECORD OF CHANGE

Documentation of the assessment of changes not in-kind and of the denial or authorization of proposed changes may be included in a form typically known as a *management record of change*. While the format for such documentation is highly variable, certain substantive information should always be included:

- potential impacts on human health and safety and on environmen-tal quality
- modifications of operating procedures required prior to implement-ing the proposed change

- scheduling requirements for implementing the proposed change
- personnel training that must be completed prior to implementing the proposed change
- any other actions required prior to or upon completion of the proposed change

Documented authorization generally includes printed names, titles, dates, and signatures of personnel having responsibility for different levels of changes. For example, the procedure depicted in Figure 14.1 requires that both the manager of the department initiating the change and the corporate safety officer sign off for any level 2 change, whereas a level 3 change requires authorization by each of the following: the manager of process development and quality assurance, the manager of engineering and maintenance, the manager of the department initiating the change, the corporate safety officer, and the plant manager.

Whatever the sign-off requirements might be, it is advisable that required signatures on the management record of change clearly indicate that all responsible individuals agree as to the assessment of the proposed change and the precautionary and follow-up requirements specified in the management record of change.

It is also advisable that, regardless of any regulatory requirements, the management record of change form, the change request form, and any other relevant information (e.g., training records) be maintained as permanent corporate records and that they be periodically reviewed (e.g., annually) as part of a continual effort to ensure the efficacy of MOC procedures.

CHAPTER 15

BLOODBORNE PATHOGENS

BACKGROUND

Bloodborne pathogens are those disease-causing (pathogenic) organisms that may be found in blood and certain other body fluids of infected persons; they may be transmitted, therefore, to other persons through contact with these fluids. The two bloodborne pathogens of primary concern are the hepatitis virus (HV), specifically types B and C (HBV and HCV, respectively), and the human immunodeficiency virus (HIV), which is really two distinct viral strains (HIV-1 and HIV-2).

HBV is of particular concern as an occupational hazard not only because it causes a long-term disabling liver disease possibly leading to cirrhosis and even liver cancer, but also because of its efficient transmission from one person to another following contact with infected blood and body fluids. HBV has caused more cases of occupationally linked infectious disease than any other bloodborne pathogen. As shown in Figure 15.1, HBV infection may require an extended period of incubation and become manifest in diverse symptoms, with many infected persons becoming long-term carriers and therefore potential sources of new infection.

In the United States, it has been estimated that on the order of 300,000 persons, including 9000 health care workers, become infected with HBV every year. Worldwide, about 300 million persons are chronic carriers of HBV; in southeast Asia and tropical Africa, chronic carriers represent at least 10% of the population; in North America and most of western Europe, less than 1%.

Historically, primary attention has been given to HBV as the primary occupationally linked hepatitis virus, while HCV (a non-A, non-B strain), which is also transmitted through blood and other body fluids, was considered to present relatively little risk in the workplace. More recently, however, HCV has been demonstrated to present potentially significant workplace

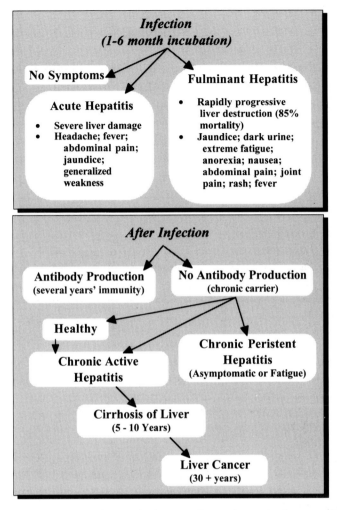

FIGURE 15.1   Alternative pathways of infection and postinfection development of HBV.

risk, with upward of 40% of hepatitis infections previously attributed to HBV now possibly attributable to HCV.

HIV is almost universally recognized as the causative agent of "Acquired Immune Deficiency Syndrome" (AIDS), a disease that contravenes the body's capacity to resist a variety of life-threatening infections. HIV infection may also lead to severe weight loss, fatigue, neurological disorders, and certain cancers, including cancer of the skin or other connective tissue (sarcoma) and cancer of the lymph nodes or lymph tissues (lymphoma).

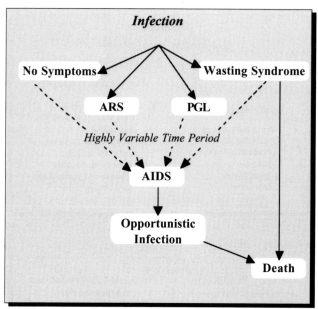

FIGURE 15.2 Alternative pathways of postinfection development of HIV (ARS, acute retroviral syndrome; PGL, persistent generalized lymphadenopathy; AIDS, acquired immunodeficiency syndrome).

First discovered in 1979, AIDS quickly attained the status of a global epidemic, with estimates of actual cases worldwide approaching 600,000 in less than a decade. While individual estimates of HIV infections or AIDS cases are always subject to much debate, all continue to indicate a persistently grim prospect, with somewhere between 38 million to 110 million adults and more than 10 million children likely infected with HIV by the year 2000 and, of these, about 24 million adults and 3 million children with fully developed AIDS—about 10 times as many as in the beginning of the current decade.

As shown in Figure 15.2, a distinction must be made between "infection with HIV" and "development of AIDS." While it must be assumed that HIV infection ultimately results in the development of AIDS, it may progress differently in different persons, both with respect to symptomatology and chronology.

One clinically distinct possibility is known as "acute retroviral syndrome" (ARS), a condition that develops within several months of exposure and which is characterized by mononucleosis-like signs and symptoms, including fever, swelling of lymph nodes, pain or tenderness in muscles and joints, diarrhea, fatigue, and rash. Another progressive condition is "persistent, generalized lymphadenopathy" (PGL), a swelling of the lymph glands that, in the absence of any other symptoms, persists for 3 or more months. It is also possible that infected persons will display no outward signs or symptoms of HIV infection at all (i.e., be asymptomatic) for months or even years.

While most infected persons do develop antibodies to HIV within 6 to 12 weeks of exposure to HIV, some may show neither outward symptoms nor an analytically detectable antibody response for even longer periods. Finally, even before the full-blown development of AIDS, which is indicated by essentially the collapse of the immune system and the subsequent development of opportunistic "indicator diseases" such as pneumonia, fungal diseases of the throat and lung, Kaposi's sarcoma, and tuberculosis, an HIV infected person may develop the "HIV wasting syndrome." This syndrome is characterized by severe, involuntary weight loss, chronic diarrhea, constant or intermittent weakness, and extended periods of fever—conditions that may themselves result in death.

Regardless of the progress of specific symptoms, and regardless of the length of time over which infected persons may remain asymptomatic, all HIV-infected persons may transmit HIV to others.

As dire as the statistics regarding HIV infection may be, it is important that the safety officer understand that the probability of infection by HBV is on the order of 100,000 times greater than the probability of infection by HIV. This is not to diminish in any way the seriousness of HIV but, rather, to emphasize that, however frightful a particular disease is, a comprehensive approach to workplace health must not be focused solely on that one disease.

In addition to HBV, HCV, and HIV, bloodborne pathogens include a variety of highly infectious agents that, despite being rare in the United States, do pose significant risk to workers in various parts of the world. As shown in Table 15.1, these pathogens include bacterial, protozoan, and viral species that, through a variety of *disease vectors*, including mosquitoes, ticks, and lice, ultimately contaminate human blood and other bodily fluids.

WORKPLACE EXPOSURE

Most frequently, the etiological and epidemiological understanding of a horrific disease lags far behind popular mythologies that thrive on long-standing personal, cultural, and national prejudices and predispositions. Thusly has both the black plague of the High Middle Ages and the current epidemic of AIDS been attributed by pretentious demagog as well as earnest demigod to godly retribution for the sinfulness of human behavior. Just what constitutes sinful behavior varies, of course, with time. Currently, it seems most often to be homosexual behavior or substance abuse. However, even

TABLE 15.1   Additional Infectious Diseases That May Be Transmitted among Humans through Contaminated Bodily Fluids

Syphilis ■➔	Sexually transmitted disease caused by the bacterial spirochete *Treponema pallidum*; most commonly transmitted by sexual contact; transmission can occur through infected blood or an open wound, or from mother to fetus; characterized by a chancre at the site of infection and by generalized eruption of the skin and mucous membranes and inflammation of eyes, bones, and central nervous system; ultimately results in chronic skin lesions, damage to the heart and aorta, and central nervous system degeneration.
Malaria ■➔	Infectious parasitic disease caused by several parasitic species of the amoeba *Plasmodium* which is transmitted through the *Anopheles* mosquito which picks up the parasite from the blood of an infected person and transfers it to that of a healthy person; characterized by high fever, severe chills, enlargement of the spleen, and sometimes anemia and jaundice.
Babesiosis ■➔	Human protozoan disease of red blood cells caused by the protozoan *Babesia microti* that is transmitted by the deer tick; characterized by fever, malaise, and hemolytic anemia; prevalent on the coastal islands of the northeast United States; also called *piroplasmosis.*
Brucellosis ■➔	An infectious bacterial disease of human beings caused by several species of *Brucella*; transmitted by contact with infected livestock or unpasteurized dairy products; characterized by fever, malaise, and headache; also called Gibraltar fever, Malta fever, Mediterranean fever, Rock fever, undulant fever.
Leptospirosis ■➔	An infectious disease of domesticated animals, including cattle, swine, and dogs; human infection due to contact with urine of infected animals; caused by bacterial spirochete *Leptospira interrogans*; characterized by jaundice and fever; also called swamp fever.
Arborviral Infections ■➔	Infections such as encephalitis, yellow fever, Colorado tick fever, and dengue fever, which are caused by a variety of viruses; transmitted by arthropods such as mosquitoes and ticks.
Relapsing Fever ■➔	Rare disease cause by bacterial spirochete *Borrelia recurrentis*; transmitted to humans by lice and ticks; characterized by chills and fever; also called recurrent fever.
Creutzfeldt - Jakob Disease ■➔	A rare, usually fatal disease of the brain; characterized by progressive dementia and gradual loss of muscle control; also called Jakob-Creutzfeldt disease. *Mad Cow Disease*
Viral Hemorrhagic Fever ■➔	A variety of infectious diseases caused by viruses; characterized by fever, chills, prostration, muscle pain, jaundice, internal hemorrhage, coma, and death.

contemporary attribution is highly diverse, sometimes defined not so much on the basis of overt behavior as on quite general circumstances, such as a person's national origin, religious affiliation, and culture.

Whatever the favorite major and minor tenets of any popular mythology regarding HIV and other bloodborne diseases, reality imposes its own rules which, regardless of personal desire, political stance, or religious conviction, pertain to all people equally:

1. Exposure to the blood and body fluids of infected persons always presents a real risk of contracting the disease—and the risk of actual exposure to infected materials cannot be lessened by any social or ethical or moral attribute of either the source of the infection or its potential new host.

2. All analytical tests devised to detect the presence of infection have inherent limits. In some instances, such limits become manifest in *false negatives*, which are analytical results that indicate that a disease is not present when it actually is present. For example, a person who is infected with HIV may nonetheless be completely asymptomatic, with blood showing no detectable levels of HIV antibody for weeks and even months after infection. The negative analytical results are therefore "false": they do *not* prove the infection is absent; they do *not* prove that the person cannot spread that infection.

3. Given the diversity of human response to infection, which may range from grossly symptomatic to completely asymptomatic, given the diverse periods of latency typically associated with the signs and symptoms of bloodborne diseases, and given inherent limits to analytical procedures performed to detect disease (e.g., false negatives or outright laboratory error), no person can safely assume that any human blood or related body fluid is not contaminated with infectious agents.

The relevance of these rules to workplace behavior and the prevention of the spread of bloodborne pathogens within and beyond the confines of the workplace is epitomized in a set of practical measures known as *Universal Precautions*.

UNIVERSAL PRECAUTIONS

Universal precautions are practices designed to prevent the transmission of bloodborne pathogens from infected to noninfected persons. The term "universal" is used to denote that these precautions must always be used when there is potential exposure to blood and other body fluids regardless of the supposed infective state of the person from which the blood or other body fluids derive. In short, under universal precautions, all persons are considered potentially infectious of HBV, HCV, HIV, and other blood-borne pathogens.

Typology of Potentially Infectious Materials

In the workplace, protection from bloodborne pathogens begins with the recognition of four basic types of potentially infectious materials:

1. Human blood, blood components, and products made from human blood
2. Human body fluids, including:

- semen (male reproductive secretion)
- vaginal secretions (female reproductive secretion)
- cerebrospinal fluid (associated with brain and spinal cord)
- synovial fluid (associated with membrane in bone joint)
- pleural fluid (associated with lung)
- pericardial fluid (associated with chest cavity)
- peritoneal fluid (associated with abdominal cavity)
- amniotic fluid (associated with membranous sack covering fetus)
- saliva (only in dental procedures, where there is a high probability of blood becoming mixed with the saliva)
- any body fluid that is visibly contaminated with blood
- all body fluids in situations where it is difficult to differentiate between body fluids

3. Any unfixed tissue or organ (other than intact skin) from a human, either living or dead (note: "unfixed" means that the tissue or organ is not chemically or physically preserved)
4. HIV- and HV-containing cultures, media, solutions, blood, organs, or other tissues from experimental animals infected with HIV or HV

The last two types of materials are of concern in a relatively restricted number of workplaces, whereas the first two pertain to all workplaces and therefore deserve special emphasis.

While universal precautions do not typically apply to feces, nasal secretions, sputum, sweat, tears, urine, and vomitus, there are many circumstances in which such materials may contain blood and other potentially infectious body fluids and therefore require universal precautions. Of course, when in doubt, it is most wise to assume that any body fluid or substance encountered in the workplace may be infectious.

Exposure-Related Workplace Activity

In a workplace that does not include the use, preparation, or analysis of human blood or other body fluids or the handling of known infectious agents, those personnel at risk of infection by bloodborne pathogens typically include:

- corporate health care personnel (e.g., company nurse, consulting physician)
- first aid providers
- emergency response personnel
- housekeeping and laundry personnel

It must be emphasized that, in any company, any person who provides aid to an injured co-worker (i.e., acts as a "good Samaritan"), regardless of job assignment, may become exposed to infectious blood or other body fluids. Types of work that routinely involve the risk of infection by bloodborne pathogens include, of course, a wide range of jobs typical of health care facilities and services, blood or disease research facilities, pharmaceutical-related work involving experimental drugs for the treatment of bloodborne pathogens, pathology laboratories, and mortuaries.

Typology of Universal Precautions

Universal precautions consist of a variety of procedures to control the risk of infection, including (a) HBV vaccination, (b) engineering controls, (c) work practice controls, and (d) personal protective equipment.

HBV Vaccination

In the United States, personnel who might become exposed to HBV in the performance of their work must be offered immunization against HBV. According to 29 CFR 1910.1030, vaccination must be offered to the at-risk worker within 10 working days of initial job assignment and at no cost to the employee. Other provisions of the OSHA regulation include:

- the vaccination is to be offered at a reasonable time and place and under the supervision of a licensed physician or a health care professional licensed to give HBV vaccinations
- an employee is not required to have a vaccination if (a) the employee has previously received the complete HBV vaccination series,

or (b) tests show the employee is immune, or (c) the vaccine is contraindicated for medical reasons
- an employee is not required to participate in a prescreening program as a prerequisite to receiving the HBV vaccination
- an employee may refuse to receive the HBV vaccination or, having initially refused, may subsequently decide to receive it

Engineering Controls

In laboratories and other production facilities that directly involve the culture, production, concentration, experimentation, and manipulation of HIV and HBV, and in facilities that routinely provide health care services, the use of isolation, physical barriers, and ventilation is a particularly important aspect of infection control. While 29 CFR 1910.1030 provides specific requirements for various types of facilities, common examples of engineering controls that are implemented as routine universal precautions include:

- physical isolation of activities involving the handling of bloodborne infectious agents, with limited and otherwise controlled entry
- the use of biological safety cabinets or other physical containment devices
- the use of leakproof containers for the storage and transport of contaminated materials
- the use of nonrecirculated directional airflow to preclude contamination of nonwork areas

Work Practice Controls

Work practice controls are those policies and procedures designed to minimize the risk of infection during the performance of routine tasks. Four basic types of work practices are relevant in any situation where exposure to bloodborne pathogens is a possibility:

1. General work practices: apply to the range of workplace tasks regardless of the type of industry

- Eating, drinking, smoking, applying cosmetics or lip balm, and wearing contact lenses should be prohibited
- Food and beverages should not be stored in cabinets, refrigerators, freezers, or on counters
- Any procedure involving blood or potentially infectious materials should be performed to minimize splashing, spraying, or the formation of droplets

- Any specimen of blood or potentially infectious material should be kept in clearly labeled, leakproof, closed containers during collection, storage, handling, processing, shipping, and transport
- Pipetting by mouth should be strictly prohibited in all circumstances
- No blood or body fluid should ever be touched or cleaned up without the use of proper protective clothing and equipment

2. The use of "sharps": practices regarding the use and disposal of needles, blades and other items that may cut or puncture the skin

- Needles or other sharps contaminated with human blood or other body fluids should not be bent, broken, sheared, recapped, or removed from holders
- Disposable sharps should be deposited in containers that are puncture-resistant, leakproof, and color coded or labeled "Biohazard"
- Nondisposable sharps should be decontaminated according to written directions

3. Accidental contact: procedures to be followed after accidental contact with human blood or other body fluids

- Immediately flush eyes with water or wash skin with soap and water
- Remove any contaminated clothing immediately and wash any areas of skin that may have been contaminated by fluids soaking through
- Obtain medical consultation after contact to determine necessity of follow-up medical treatment or prophylaxis

4. Housekeeping: procedures governing the clean-up of spills of blood and body fluids, as well as general housekeeping tasks

- Housekeeping personnel should be trained in proper techniques for cleaning any spill of blood or potentially infectious materials, including the use of personal protective equipment and disinfectants
- All blood-soaked rags and papers should be placed in biohazard bags, sealed, and disposed of through a biohazard-certified (medical waste) facility
- Contaminated linens and other laundry should be sealed in biohazard bags and the laundry service notified of the potential for exposure
- Trash receptacles in areas where contamination is likely should be cleaned and decontaminated immediately following any contamination

- All areas contaminated by blood or other body fluids should be decontaminated

Personal Protective Clothing and Equipment

Whenever engineering and work practice controls are inadequate for preventing exposure, personal protective equipment and clothing should be used.

- Disposable vinyl or latex gloves should be used wherever hand contact with bloodborne pathogens may occur
- An emergency packet should be immediately available to emergency responders and other personnel who may become exposed to bloodborne pathogens and should contain (a) disposable vinyl or latex gloves, (b) appropriate disinfectant solution, (c) a supply of absorbent containment material and scoop, (d) biohazard bags, and (e) disposable towels (for stanching copious flows of blood without exposing responders to blood splash)
- Disposable gloves must not be cleaned or washed for reuse; however, they should be cleaned prior to removal and disinfected following removal or discarded into biohazard bags
- No petroleum products (e.g., hand creams) should be used in conjunction with latex gloves because such materials may degrade latex
- Under no circumstances should mouth-to-mouth resuscitation be performed; protective mouthpieces or ambu bags should be used to prevent contact with potentially blood-contaminated saliva
- Additional protective clothing should be provided as circumstances may require, including fluidproof aprons, goggles, shoe covers, and face shields

EXPOSURE CONTROL PLAN

Under the provisions of 29 CFR 1910.1030, the employer must develop a written exposure control plan (ECP). The specific objectives of this plan are (a) to designate job classifications that present the risk of exposure to bloodborne pathogens, (b) to define the schedule and means for implementing exposure controls, and (c) to establish procedures for the evaluation of exposure incidents, personnel training, and record-keeping.

The regulations provide specific guidance regarding those work-related activities that may result in exposure to bloodborne pathogens:

1. Job categories in which all employees in those categories have potential occupational exposure (e.g., nurses, physicians, first-aid providers)

2. Job categories in which some employees in those categories have potential occupational exposure (e.g., laundry workers, housekeeping personnel)

3. Individual tasks and procedures or groups of closely related tasks and procedures in which some or all employees may experience exposure to bloodborne pathogens (e.g., emergency responders, members of a fire brigade)

In addition to these criteria, every company must consider the potential for exposure of the good Samaritan—a role, after all, that may be played by any employee, both in and outside of the workplace.

Many companies address the potential exposure of the good Samaritan by ensuring that all personnel receive training in the risks attendant to exposure to human blood and body fluids and in basic precautions that should always be taken when providing first-aid. In many instances, companies establish written policies that are intended to exempt personnel from any job-related requirement to play the role of the good Samaritan. However, it must be said that such policies are of dubious legal value and, in the absence of any corporate effort to provide personnel with timely access to appropriate protective equipment and materials and proper training, of highly questionable ethical value. The best way to control exposure of the good Samaritan is to ensure that all employees have immediate access to protective equipment and materials and know how to use them. The capital investment in protective equipment and training is, by any measure, trivial and should be considered a standard expense in any business.

Among the various procedures to be implemented regarding the control of exposure to bloodborne pathogens, particular attention must be given to oversight and enforcement. It cannot be overemphasized that the protection of workers who might become exposed to bloodborne pathogens and other body fluids means protection from infections that can easily spread beyond the workplace into workers' families and the community at large. This broad social responsibility for the control of disease means that compliance with workplace policies and procedures designed to control severely disabling and even life-threatening disease must be rigorously enforced without exception.

Special attention must also be given to those procedures regarding the evaluation of any incident of workplace exposure, especially the methodical and detailed assessment of any related failures with regard to the identification of jobs and personnel at risk, the adequacy of engineering and work practice controls, personal protective clothing and equipment, and personnel training. Each postexposure incident evaluation should include specific recommendations for revising the exposure control plan as well as precise schedules for implementing those revisions and monitoring their effectiveness.

PART III

SPECIAL ISSUES

CHAPTER 16

CHEMICAL SURVEILLANCE AND MONITORING

SCOPE

Today, chemical surveillance of the workplace is standard practice, with specific requirements defined not only by regulatory authority (e.g., emergency response, laboratory standard, confined space entry, respiratory protection, hazard communication, or chemical process safety) but also by corporate insurance carriers, corporate legal counsel, health and safety professionals, and by employees themselves. It is, in fact, as intrinsic to modern business practice as loss control, total quality management and human resource development.

Given the broad legal, political, economic, and ethical ramifications of exposure to workplace chemicals, it is useful to distinguish between "chemical monitoring" and "chemical surveillance."

Chemical monitoring connotes the technical and methodological aspects of any qualitative or quantitative analysis of process or fugitive chemicals. It may be undertaken for a variety of reasons, including not only the management of potential human exposures, but also to control production processes or the quality of intermediate and finished products. Chemical surveillance is a much broader, programmatic approach to the management of human exposure to chemicals. Surveillance includes monitoring, but also includes a variety of other efforts, such as the control of chemical inventories, waste minimization, chemical substitution, and process management.

CHEMICAL MONITORING TECHNOLOGY

Common techniques for monitoring workplace chemicals that present human health and safety risks may be conveniently divided into three basic types:

1. Ambient air monitoring: techniques that provide relatively rapid on-site detection or measurement of chemicals that are present in the air as dusts, vapors, or mists,
2. Ambient materials testing: techniques that typically require off-site laboratory analysis of samples, including solids (e.g., soil samples) and liquids (e.g., groundwater, tap water, mixtures of waste), and
3. Personal monitoring: techniques that involve the detection or measurement of chemicals (a) within body tissues such as blood or urine or (b) in the immediate vicinity of a worker equipped with a personal monitor to measure cumulative exposure over a specific period of time.

Ambient Air Monitoring Devices

By far the most common chemical monitoring devices used in industry, these devices provide a rapid, direct reading of chemical concentrations in air. However, there are usually significant limitations associated with any particular device, including the following:

- most detect or measure only specific chemicals or chemical classes; none detect all possible chemicals
- while the sensitivity of such devices is always subject to the development of new technology, they are generally incapable of detecting airborne concentrations of chemicals below 1 mg/liter (ppm)
- many can give false readings because, although designed to detect one particular substance, they are subject to interference by the presence of other chemicals

Colorimetric Indicator Tube

This relatively low-priced and easily used device consists of (a) a tubular glass ampoule containing an "indicator chemical" that reacts with a specific ambient contaminant of interest and (b) a manual or motorized pump to draw a calibrated amount of ambient air through the ampoule. The reaction of the indicator chemical and the air contaminant changes the color of the indicator chemical; the linear length of the color change in the ampoule is proportional to the concentration of the air contaminant. Calculating the air concentration of the contaminant requires a simple mathematical operation involving the calibrated length of the color reaction in the ampoule and the volume of air pumped through the device; depending upon the specific chemical being measured, the calculation may also require correction for barometric pressure. The measurement of certain air contaminants may also

TABLE 16.1 Data and Information Typically Provided by Manufacturers of Colorimetric Devices Used for the Monitoring of Common Industrial Chemicals

Gas or vapor to be monitored	Catalog number	Range (ppm/ hours)	Detection limit (ppm; 8-hour)	Color change	Storage temp.	Shelf-life (years)
Ammonia	3D	25–500 ppm	1.0	Purple to yellow	Room temp.	3
Carbon dioxide	2D	0.2–8.0% hr.	0.015%	Blue to white	Room temp.	2
Carbon monoxide	1D	50–1000 ppm	2.5	Yellow to dark brown	Room temp.	2
Chlorine	8D	2–50 ppm	0.13	White to yellow	Room temp.	2
Formaldehyde	91D	1–20 ppm	0.06	Yellow to red brown	Refrigerate	1
Hydrogen cyanide	12D	10–200 ppm	0.5	Orange to red	Room temp.	2
Hydrogen sulfide	4D	10–200 ppm	0.25	White to dark brown	Room temp.	3
Nitrogen dioxide	9D	1–30 ppm	0.06	White to yellow	Refrigerate	1
Sulfur dioxide	5D	5–100 ppm	0.13	Green to yellow	Room temp.	2

require the simultaneous use of a second ampoule, which is affixed to the indicator tube.

Manufacturers of colorimetric indicator tubes provide detailed information on the limits of each indicator tube that is specific to the ambient gas or vapor of interest (Table 16.1). In addition to such chemical-specific limitations, all colorimetric tubes share certain general limitations:

- while each indicator tube is specific to a particular ambient chemical, other ambient contaminants can interfere with the indicator chemical
- most tubes can be affected by high humidity, thereby giving false readings
- tubes available from different manufacturers may have different sensitivities, thereby providing different measurements of ambient concentrations
- because of the variability of color perception among persons, different personnel may make different judgments as to the length of the color stain within the indicator ampoule

Another common problem associated with colorimetric indicator devices is the problem of "false negatives." If, after use, an ampoule shows no color reaction, the negative result may be due to (a) the concentration of the ambient contaminant being lower than the sensitivity of the tube or (b) the indicator tube being defective. In such a case, the user is well advised to test the negative ampoule with a known high concentration of the contaminant vapor.

Finally, it must be stressed that the volume of air perfused through the indicator tube is typically very small and therefore represents a very tiny portion of the ambient air. The location of the air intake to the detection device is therefore critical with regard to estimating air quality in the volume of air actually breathed by employees. It is always advisable to conduct colorimetric monitoring within the immediate breathing space of the employee at possible risk. High flow personal samplers are increasingly available and should be considered as an important adjunct to any monitoring program. Single pumps are typically housed in a lightweight plastic case which clips to the user's belt. Multiple pumps are also available and can be used for simultaneous monitoring of atmospheric samples taken at different locations within the same general area. Battery packs for both single and multiple samplers allow continuous sampling over an 8- to 10-hr period.

Electronic Devices

A wide range of electronic devices are available for the detection of specific chemicals and broad categories of chemicals. Some, such as the combustible gas indicator, flame ionization detector, portable infrared spectrophotometer, and ultraviolet photoionization detector (Table 16.2), have broad application for compliance with numerous health and safety regulations, including those pertaining to hazard communication, laboratory safety, emergency response, and hazardous waste. Others, such as an oxygen meter (e.g., confined space regulations) or sound meter (e.g., noise regulations), are mandated primarily by individual regulations.

Increasingly available today are electronic instruments that combine monitoring capabilities for different chemicals. Examples of such combined capabilities include:

- a combustible gas meter that also measures oxygen, hydrogen sulfide, and carbon monoxide
- a toxic gas meter that can detect oxygen and combustible gases and which can also be equipped to monitor hydrogen cyanide, hydrogen chloride, nitrogen dioxide, nitrous oxide, and sulfur dioxide
- a hazardous gas detector that gives continuous measurements of many gases, including acetone, ammonia, arsine, benzene, carbon monoxide, ethylene oxide, and formaldehyde

Of critical importance in any company that uses, handles, or stores flammable or combustible chemicals is the combustible gas indicator, which

TABLE 16.2 Basic Types of Electronic Monitoring Devices[a]

Combustible Gas Indicator (CGI)

- Measures the concentration of a combustible gas or vapor
- A filament, usually made of platinum, is heated by burning the combustible gas or vapor; the increase in heat is measured
- Accuracy depends, in part, on the difference between the calibration and sampling temperatures
- Sensitivity is a function of the differences in the chemical and physical properties between the calibration gas and the gas being sampled
- The filament can be damaged by certain compounds, such as silicones, halides, tetraethyl lead and oxygen-enriched atmospheres

Flame Ionization Detector (FID) with Gas Chromatography Option

- In "survey mode," detects the total concentrations of many organic gases and vapors; all the organic compounds are ionized and detected at the same time
- In "GC mode," identifies and measures specific compounds; volatile species are separated
- Gases and vapors are ionized in a flame; a current is produced in proportion to the number of carbon atoms present
- Does not detect inorganic gases and vapors, or some synthetics; sensitivity depends on the compound
- Should not be used at temperatures < 40 deg. F (4 deg. C)
- Difficult to identify compounds absolutely; specific identification requires calibration with the specific compound of interest
- High concentrations of contaminants or oxygen-deficient atmospheres require system modification
- In "survey mode," readings can only be reported relative to the calibration standard used

Portable Infrared (IR) Spectrophotometer

- Measures concentration of many gases and vapors in air
- Passes different frequencies of IR through the sample; the frequencies absorbed are specific for each compound
- In the field, must make repeated passes to achieve reliable results
- Not approved for use in a potentially flammable or explosive atmosphere
- Water vapor and carbon dioxide interfere with detection
- Certain vapors and high moisture may attach to the instrument's optics, which must then be replaced

Ultraviolet (UV) Photoionization Detector (PID)

- Detects total concentrations of many organic and some inorganic gases and vapors; some identification of compounds is possible if more than one probe is used
- Ionizes molecules using UV radiation; produces a current that is proportional to the number of ions
- Does not detect a compound if the probe used has a lower energy level than the compound's ionization potential
- Response may change when gases are mixed
- Other voltage sources may interfere with measurements; response is affected by high humidity

[a] Adapted from materials provided by NIOSH, OSHA, U.S. Coast Guard, and U.S. EPA.

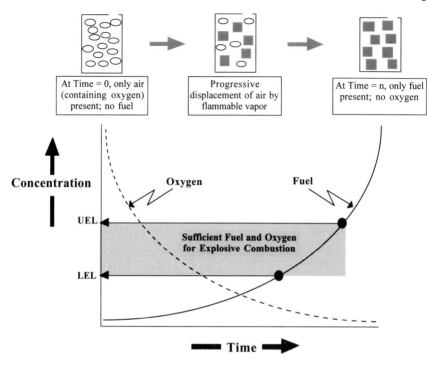

FIGURE 16.1 Lower and upper explosive limits. As the air in a container is progressively displaced by a flammable vapor (upper portion of figure), the concentration of oxygen in the container decreases while the concentration of potential fuel increases. At concentrations of fuel (expressed as percentage of atmosphere) below the LEL (lower explosive limit), there is too little fuel to support burning; at concentrations of fuel above the UEL (upper explosive limit), there is too little oxygen to support burning. Explosion may occur only when the relative concentrations of fuel and oxygen are at or between the LEL and UEL. On a scale where 100% represents the LEL, 10% is typically used as the trigger for implementing personnel evacuation.

usually measures the lower explosive limit of a combustible gas or vapor in terms of lower explosive limit. As depicted in Figure 16.1, the combustion of a substance depends upon an adequate supply of both burnable fuel and oxygen.

The relative amounts of oxygen and fuel that will support combustion can be described in terms of the *lower explosive limit* (LEL) and *upper explosive limit* (UEL). Below the LEL, there is insufficient fuel to support combustion; above the UEL, there is insufficient oxygen. The readout of the combustion meter is typically in terms of "percentage of LEL," with 100% indicating that the mixture of fuel and oxygen meets the minimal requirement for explosion. On such a scale, a reading of 10%, which is increasingly used to trigger the evacuation of an area, means that the concentration of flammable vapor in that area is 1/10th of that required for a state of imminent explosion.

Portable detectors (Table 16.2) can, with proper calibration, detect hundreds of individual toxic vapors and gases. FID (flame ionization dector) and PID (photoionization detector) units can also be operated to measure total concentrations of ambient chemicals without regard to individual chemical species. This mode of operation (often called survey mode) is useful because its lack of chemical specificity provides an inherent safety factor. For example, in the survey mode, a reading of, say, 250 ppm, which could represent a total concentration of potentially hundreds of organic compounds, could also be interpreted to represent the concentration of a particularly toxic compound of concern. Such a worst-case interpretation of the reading might or might not be realistic in a particular circumstance, but such an interpretation always has very real value as a criterion for further investigatory (if not corrective) action.

An oxygen meter (and, in some circumstances, a toxic gas and/or combustible gas meter), is a basic requirement in any workplace containing confined spaces. While there are many different designs of oxygen meters, it is imperative that the meter be provided with a long probe that can be lowered or otherwise extended into a confined space without the operator becoming exposed to an atmosphere that is potentially oxygen deficient. It is also important that the operator understand that an oxygen meter is highly sensitive to various factors, including barometric pressure and ambient concentrations of carbon dioxide and other oxidizing agents (e.g., ozone).

In this regard, it must be stressed that, despite their apparent simplicity of design and operation, all electronic detectors are sophisticated instruments and require a precise understanding of their inherent limitations and requirements regarding calibration, care, and maintenance. The safety officer is well advised to ensure that the manufacturer of any electronic detector provides on site instruction of personnel in all aspects of operation and maintenance of these devices, with particular emphasis given to the routine documentation of calibration, precision, and accuracy.

Ambient Materials Testing

In many situations a safety officer may require analyses of materials that cannot be performed on site, such as the analysis of:

- potable water supplies in the workplace, including wells, public water supply mains and lines, and workplace bubblers or taps, which might be contaminated with biological or chemical materials
- surface or groundwater supplies that might become contaminated by corporate or off-site activities and present health or safety risks to employees or the general public

- on-site soils and dusts possibly contaminated with heavy metals
- structural and other on-site materials containing toxic substances (e.g., asbestos, pesticide residues, lead based paint)

Such analyses typically require the use of specialized laboratories, including commercial water testing laboratories and materials testing laboratories. Where such professional analytical services are required, the safety officer should select those vendors who are certified by legal authority—and, more precisely, those who are specifically certified for the particular analysis to be performed. For example, in the United States a water testing laboratory may be certified through a state agency under the aegis of the U.S. Environmental Protection Agency—however, the certification is typically highly specific on the basis of the different types of analyses required by the Federal Safe Drinking Water Act, with certification for the analysis of heavy metals, for example, being separate and distinct from certification for the analysis of microorganisms.

Having procured the professional services of an appropriately certified laboratory, the safety officer must ensure that all samples are collected, stored, and delivered in full compliance with relevant regulations. In all instances, it is desirable that the contracted certified laboratory itself collect and handle samples. Where this is not possible, the safety officer should obtain written directions from the certified laboratory for the proper procedure for collecting, handling, packaging, preserving, transporting, and documenting samples.

Personal Monitoring

Personal monitoring devices include as "badges," "monitors," "dosimeters," and "diffusion detector tubes," all of which can easily be clipped or otherwise attached to personal clothing (e.g., pockets, labels). Monitors may be dedicated to a particular chemical species (e.g., mercury vapor, trichloroethylene) or provide detection of broad classes of chemicals (e.g., organic vapors). In some designs, monitors that detect classes of chemicals may be processed to yield specific exposure data regarding a limited number of specific chemicals out of several dozen possibilities. Some devices give direct readouts of a timed exposure or require simple comparison of color changes with standard color charts or data sheets; others require off-site laboratory processing, which introduces delays of several or more days in obtaining data.

Because of the necessary delays in obtaining data from badges that require off-site processing, it is imperative that such devices not be used when an 8-hr workplace exposure can exceed safety standards, including 8-hr, short-term (e.g., 15-min) or "immediately dangerous to life" (IDLH) values. The basic rule is that personal monitoring devices be used only after a comprehensive survey of the workplace has established, by means of ambient monitoring devices, potential worst-case exposures. Personal monitoring devices may then be selected to ensure that workers do not become, in effect, "canaries" that, despite a sense of safety imparted by the technical sophistication of their personal monitors, abruptly signal a hazardous situation by dying.

PROGRAMMATIC APPROACH TO MONITORING

No monitoring should be undertaken except as part of any overall surveillance program that has been designed with meticulous attention to the following considerations:

Identification of Parameters

The key requirements for including any parameter in a monitoring program are: (a) that a consensual health or safety standard for the parameter exists and (b) that the proposed monitoring technique or device for measuring that parameter is accepted by regulatory authority or by the broad scientific community. The safety officer is advised to distinguish between "proposed" and "acceptable" health and safety standards and analytical methodologies. Toward this end, the safety officer must be thoroughly familiar with jurisdictionally relevant health and safety regulations, which typically specify both the appropriate interpretative standard (e.g., maximum concentration level) and the appropriate methodological standard (i.e., analytical technique).

Baseline Concentrations

The concentration of ambient chemicals in the workplace typically varies greatly over the a workday. Before any schedule of ambient monitoring or sampling is established, it is necessary to conduct a baseline study to identify the range of variation that may be correlated with routine workplace production schedules, seasonal patterns of temperature and humidity (which may directly influence in-plant ventilation), and plant production levels. A baseline study must also note variations in ambient concentrations of chemicals with regard to nonroutine situations, as in the case of power outages and staged shutdowns of ventilation for equipment repair or replacement.

Frequency of Monitoring

Too often the frequency of monitoring is determined on the basis of arbitrary judgments of "reasonableness" rather than objective management-based criteria. For example, a company may decide to monitor all flammable cabinets with a combustion meter once every 6 months—a decision that may be eminently reasonable in terms of personnel constraints. However, such a schedule may also be judged to be totally irrelevant if it can be demonstrated that the variation in dangerous levels of combustible vapors has a periodicity of several days or weeks or that the periodicity of critical concentrations varies from one cabinet to another, depending on nonlinear work loads.

The point is that no schedule for monitoring can be predetermined by any arbitrary factor; the frequency of monitoring can be determined only by the need to detect variations in concentrations that lie beyond the limits established by the baseline study. It is, after all, to be assumed that all in-place precautionary efforts, including engineering and work practice controls as well as personal protective equipment, are predicated on data obtained from the baseline study. The objective of monitoring is, *first*, to detect any aberrations from baseline conditions, *second*, to use such aberrations to trigger additional protective and corrective action and, *third*, to revise continually the description of baseline conditions on the basis of aberrations observed as a result of ongoing monitoring.

Action Levels

Some regulations (e.g., 29 CFR 1910, subpart Z) specify actions to be taken if monitoring data regarding certain chemicals (e.g., formaldehyde) meet or exceed certain limits called *action levels*. While the number of chemicals having action levels defined by legal regulations is small, the key requirement for any monitoring program is that corporate action levels be defined for all monitored parameters.

In the typical situation, routine monitoring data are collected, recorded, and, over some period of time involving days, weeks, and months, processed and eventually filed. Oftentimes, the employee who conducts the monitoring is not the employee responsible for reviewing the data. This approach is in direct opposition to the objective of using monitoring data to ensure the health and safety of personnel. Persons who conduct the monitoring and have first access to the resultant data must be equipped with clear criteria for immediately initiating any action that must be taken in consequence of those data. Data that meet or exceed established action levels are not to be used to "call a meeting" to discuss the ramifications of the data. They must trigger immediate action to protect personnel and to correct a hazardous situation—actions that have already been assessed and fully formulated.

Notification

It is increasingly recognized throughout modern business that workers have the right of access to any information regarding their workplace exposure to hazardous chemicals. In the United States, workers' rights regarding workplace exposure are specifically addressed not only within regulations that focus on individual categories of hazards, but also in 29 CFR 1910.20, which generally applies to employee exposure and medical records. At the minimum, employees should know how to find out which parameters are included in a corporate monitoring program, how the monitoring is to be conducted, and what the data pertaining to their own exposures mean in terms of their own health and safety. Copies of personal monitoring data should always be readily available to the employee's physician.

"Carry-Home" Contamination

Most often overlooked in corporate monitoring programs is the contamination that may be carried home or elsewhere from the workplace by hair, clothes, shoes, and other personal items. Even where the company attempts to control such carry-home contamination by the use of site-restricted shop uniforms and specifically required workplace practices (workplace showers, hair nets, etc.), it is advisable to consider the potential inclusion of personal clothing and other items in a comprehensive monitoring program. Even where the potential for such carry-home contamination is negligible, periodic monitoring data can provide documentation that might prove important in a legal proceeding involving any claim of corporate negligence related to chemical health and safety. Such data are also important in setting contractual responsibilities with company out-service contractors, including corporate laundry and vehicle maintenance services.

Oversight and Quality Control

In addition to routinely scheduled monitoring activities, the safety officer is well advised to consider implementing unscheduled or even randomized monitoring efforts. Such unscheduled monitoring, whether conducted by in-plant personnel or external consultants, is a potentially useful means of ensuring the adequacy of routine monitoring in terms of both programmatic scope and performance.

THE ALARP PRINCIPLE

While regulatory standards must always inform and guide any program of in-plant monitoring and surveillance, the objective of keeping workplace ambient concentrations of chemical contaminants "as low as reasonably practicable" (ALARP) is internationally recognized as a universally relevant objective. Elevated to a principle within a globally competitive business community, ALARP properly emphasizes that regulatory standards should be considered maximum allowable limits. However, within those regulatory limits, the company should endeavor to set action levels for monitoring data that minimize all workplace exposures to hazardous chemicals and other agents within the constraints of available technology and economic reasonableness.

In formulating a program of workplace monitoring that is consistent with ALARP, companies are well advised to consider that, notwithstanding the necessity of employing standard health and safety standards as well as standard analytical techniques and devices, specific technological and economic criteria for setting action levels are assessed in terms of what the "best" companies actually do.

CHAPTER 17

MEDICAL SURVEILLANCE

Medical surveillance has become an intrinsic activity in any modern workplace. Various interrelated factors are responsible, including extensive public awareness of workplace health and safety risks, engendered by the explosion of telecommunication technology; the increased exposure of corporations and corporate executives to potential liability regarding the exposure of both employees and the general public to workplace chemicals; continually expansive regulatory requirements at all levels of government; and the rapid development of a global economy in which the protection of human health is rapidly becoming a basic precept of highly competitive marketing.

While the nature and extent of medical surveillance in the workplace are variable with legal jurisdiction and type of industry, the broad dimensions of contemporary workplace medical surveillance are clearly established. Typically, medical surveillance may be subdivided into four basic categories: preemployment screening, periodic operational monitoring, episodic monitoring, and termination examination.

PREEMPLOYMENT SCREENING

Preemployment screening typically encompasses three objectives:

- to determine the fitness of an employee to perform assigned work
- to identify any health conditions that might exacerbate workplace hazards
- to establish a baseline health profile that can be used to measure the effects of subsequent workplace exposures

While each of these objectives is essential to the protection of workers, each is increasingly the subject of concern regarding a potential abasement of workers' rights—especially in light of the possible use of sophisticated clinical and genetic analyses to deny or otherwise restrict employment on the basis of potential health care costs likely to be borne by the employer. It has become clear that the increasingly widespread use over the last decade of the "temporary employee," who is typically ineligible for health care and other work-related benefits, may well reflect a pervasive corporate intent to disclaim any long-term financial responsibility for worker health rather than simply to improve cost efficiency by reducing in-house staffs devoted to employee recruitment and training. There can be little doubt that the use of preemployment screening as a means of disenfranchising the employee-at-risk rather than as a means of protecting that employee will long continue to be the focus of legal, political, and social scrutiny and debate.

Medical surveillance undertaken to determine fitness for work must be predicated on a precise understanding of the total range of health and safety hazards associated with individual work assignments, including routine and emergency requirements, as well as pertinent regulatory requirements (e.g., medical examination for use of respirator). While primarily defined by job requirements, fitness for work must also be determined in terms of any preexisting health conditions or limitations of the worker—a determination that may often be at odds with the desires of both the worker and the employer. The employer is well advised that the willingness of a worker to undertake risks contrary to professional medical advice generally does not abrogate the employer's responsibility for the health and safety of that worker. This fact underscores the importance of implementing a medical surveillance program that not only complies with the requirements of pertinent occupational health and safety regulations but also the constraints and limitations imposed by corporate legal counsel.

Of critical importance in any medical surveillance program is the establishment of baseline health profiles of at-risk employees. The comparison of these profiles with the results of subsequent surveillance is the basic means for detecting changes in health that may be related to routine and nonroutine workplace exposures. It is therefore essential that the medical examination performed in preemployment screening include those measurements of vital signs, vision and hearing measurements, lung function tests, and other clinical biochemical analyses that are directly relevant to subsequent workplace exposures. The selection of specific tests and analyses and the type of data and information required must be made only with the professional advice of a competent medical authority who is provided with all in-plant details regarding potential routine and emergency workplace exposures. The medical surveillance program must, therefore, be understood to be facility-specific; no guideline can be provided for identifying the specific tests and analyses to be included in a surveillance program that is universally appropriate throughout industry.

PERIODIC OPERATIONAL MONITORING

The sole objective of periodic operational monitoring is the early detection of adverse health effects of routine exposures to hazardous agents. As discussed above, periodic operational monitoring must be integrally linked with the baseline profiles established during preemployment screening. In designing the operational monitoring program, the safety officer should pay particular attention to the following issues:

1. Because of the wide diversity in types of hazardous agents, the variable progression of different kinds of health impairments and conditions, and the range of workplace exposures, it is highly unlikely that a monitoring schedule appropriate for the early detection of one kind of health condition will be appropriate for the early detection of another kind. For example, depending upon specific workplace conditions, an annual schedule for blood testing to detect liver disease may not be appropriate for chest X-rays, which may cause lung injury if used too frequently.

2. Differences noted between baseline profiles and subsequent operational monitoring do not necessarily indicate an actual disease or debilitation; even where a disease or debilitation is detected, it is not necessarily due to workplace exposure. All medical monitoring data and information are subject to normal variation; abnormal results that may indicate disease or debilitation may reflect home and recreational exposures as well as workplace exposures to hazardous agents. The design of an operational monitoring program must therefore be undertaken with a clear understanding of statistical and other criteria of significance that medical professionals must use when interpreting monitoring results. It is strongly recommended that personnel included in a medical surveillance program be provided with documentation regarding these criteria.

3. A properly designed medical surveillance program should include a detailed "action plan" that precisely describes steps to be taken whenever operational monitoring results in the detection of a medically significant condition, including follow-up medical examinations, tests, and treatments. The action plan should also provide for the implementation of a comprehensive in-plant review of operations, conditions, and procedures that may have contributed to the detected health impairment and which may be corrected.

EPISODIC MONITORING

Episodic medical monitoring includes any *nonroutine* medical monitoring or surveillance activity undertaken in response to a specific incident or emergency condition, such as a chemical spill, fire, or explosion or employee complaints of unusual health symptoms (e.g., persistent headaches or nausea, fainting spells). While episodic monitoring is specifically addressed in certain regulations (e.g., 29 CFR 1910.1450; 29 CFR 1910.120), it is appropriately included in any comprehensive medical surveillance program, regardless of regulatory jurisdiction.

Provision for episodic medical monitoring must be predicated on several considerations:

1. While the episode that triggers nonroutine medical surveillance may often be described in terms of objective criteria, such as an actual chemical spill or fire, subjective criteria may alone be sufficient and even critical. Even in the absence of any objectively manifest evidence of exposure, the fact that employees think they may have suffered a nonroutine exposure is sufficient cause for medical surveillance and consultation over and above any surveillance and consultation provided by regularly scheduled operational monitoring.

While many safety officers are—sometimes, with good reason—apt to consider an individual complaint the product of an overactive imagination or the purposeful contrivance of a "problem employee," safety officers are reminded that individual employees may be particularly sensitive to a hazardous agent. Should a complaint be ignored simply because it is the complaint of a single person, it is possible that a real health threat will be ignored—with not only dire consequence to that individual, but also serious legal and financial ramifications for both the company and the safety officer.

2. Whatever the cause or circumstance of the episode, medical authority must be provided with relevant data and information. In many instances, companies use standard forms to inform medical professionals of relevant information (Figure 17.1). In all instances, it is necessary that preliminary liaison be established between the safety officer and medical personnel so that the latter have direct access to baseline information that may become relevant to any subsequent episode. Such baseline information should at a minimum include a chemical inventory that, for each listed chemical, identifies hazards, target organs, and routes of entry. It is also recommended that combustion products be identified for each chemical included in the inventory, along with the hazards and target organs associated with those combustion products.

3. Episodic events that trigger medical surveillance include those defined by the recognition of health symptoms. It is therefore essential that all personnel receive thorough training in the range of symptoms that may be associated with workplace exposure to hazardous agents and understand the importance of reporting such symptoms to corporate authority.

As shown in Table 17.1, symptoms associated with exposure to hazardous agents in the workplace cannot be differentiated from symptoms associated with exposure to hazardous agents outside the workplace or from

---

Global Enterprises, Inc.

Personnel Exposure Determination Form

Employee Identification

Name

[ ]

Department

[ ]

Reason for Implementing Determination of Exposure

[ ] Monitoring Data
[ ] Observed Spill or Release of Chemical
[ ] Odor, Taste or Other Sensory Perception of Chemical
[ ] Procedural/Operational Potential (e.g., open vessel; failure of ventilation)
[ ] Signs or Symptoms of Chemical Exposure

Name(s) of Chemicals or Chemical Constituents and Relevant OSHA TLV

Chemical Name   OSHA TLV

_____   _____
_____   _____
_____   _____
_____   _____

Available Monitoring Data

Chemical Name   Date   Value/Unit

_____   _____   _____
_____   _____   _____
_____   _____   _____
_____   _____   _____

Description of Incident or Circumstance

_____   _____
Date   Signature of Safety Officer

FIGURE 17.1 Example of a corporate form that provides an attending physician or other medical professional with critical information regarding personnel exposure to a hazardous chemical.

various health conditions or infections totally unrelated to the workplace. However, the safety officer must understand that the only competent authority for determining the significance of any health symptom is the physician. It is the responsibility of the physician to evaluate symptoms and to

TABLE 17.1   Common Symptoms That May Indicate Exposure to Hazardous Chemicals[a]

Chest pain or discomfort
Bluish lips or face; extreme paleness
Persistent coughing or sneezing
Breathing discomfort; rapid or strained breathing
Palpitations or fluttering in chest
Lightheadedness or dizziness; giddiness; fainting
Headaches (especially persistent, recurrent or progressive)
Itching or irritation of eye; watering of eye; sensitivity to light
Visual impairment, including reduced vision, double vision and changes in perception of color
Loss of physical coordination or dexterity; slurring of speech
Unusual hair loss
Bleeding of gums or nose
Increased sensitivity to noise; changes in hearing acuity; ringing in ears
Abnormal odor of breath
Hoarseness
Fever
Abnormal sweating or dryness of skin
Generalized aches and pains; muscle cramping; weakness of a particular muscle
Prickly sensation in legs, arms, or face
Prickly or numb sensation in tongue
Nausea, vomiting, abdominal pain; burning sensation in throat or stomach
Unusual thirst
Problems in swallowing; change in taste sensation
Loss of appetite
Changes in color of urine
Unusual skin rashes or swelling; acne-like skin lesions; blisters
Changes in skin color
Personality changes
Abrupt or progressive behavioral changes, including changes in personal grooming; impair-
   ment of judgment; aggressiveness; irritability
Nervousness or restlessness; tremors or shakes
Lethargy or unusual sleepiness

[a] Adapted from materials provided by Dr. Donald G. Erickson.

determine the relevance of those symptoms to workplace conditions; it is the responsibility of the safety officer (and the company) to ensure that the employee who displays health symptoms has immediate access to the physician.

4. As important as symptoms are for triggering medical consultation and surveillance, the limitations of symptoms must be recognized. For example, the health effects of exposure to many hazardous chemicals often require years and decades to develop. In such cases, there may be no readily recognized symptoms for extended periods of time, whereas in others, clear symptoms develop rapidly after exposure to the hazardous agent (Figure 17.2). In compiling a list of symptoms requiring corporate notification, the safety officer must therefore ensure consideration of the range of symp-

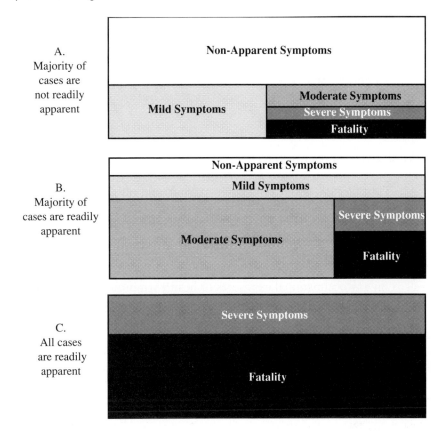

FIGURE 17.2 Distribution of clinical severity for three distinct types of infection. Other distributional patterns are possible, depending upon the specific infection.

toms associated with both chronic and acute health effects. It is also necessary to identify which particular symptoms require immediate emergency response action.

The inherent limitation of symptomatology as a trigger to medical consultation means that the safety officer must also establish additional triggering criteria, including (but not limited to):

- Fire or explosion, which may result in exposure of personnel not only to raw feedstock chemicals, but also their combustion products
- Accidental spill or release of hazardous liquids, gases, fumes, vapors, and dusts, including by-products of production processes, maintenance, or other operational activities

- Power failures that may result in failure of ventilation systems, with possible release of hazardous fumes into nonprotected areas
- Temperature inversions or other atmospheric phenomena that result in the in-plant entrainment of hazardous vapors or dusts
- Unexplained losses in stored chemicals or supplies, which may include losses due to slow and unobserved leaks or seepage of hazardous materials

TERMINATION EXAMINATION

The objective of the termination examination is to complete the total health profile of the employee over the full period of employment. While specific requirements may be defined by pertinent regulations (e.g., 29 CFR 1910.120) or, more commonly, by corporate insurance underwriters, the termination examination must be based on preemployment screening, operational, and episodic monitoring data and information available to date as well as on any occupational exposures or health symptoms experienced between the last medical examination and the termination examination.

In addition to the taking of specimens for the purpose of conducting final clinical or biochemical analyses (e.g., urinalysis, blood count, enzymes), it is possible that companies will increasingly request specimens to be warehoused for potential future analyses by as yet undeveloped or currently experimental methodologies. Such an approach, which is now rarely practiced, will most likely receive increased attention due to mutually enforcing trends in rapidly expanding analytical technologies and in workplace health and safety litigation.

LIAISON WITH MEDICAL AUTHORITIES

The various types of information and data generated in the progress of medical consultation and examination may be described in somewhat different terms by different medical practitioners and measured by different methodologies. For example, a "physical examination" given by any physician typically varies greatly from one physician to another, especially with regard to the physician's focus on a person's overall health as opposed to a focus on health in terms of workplace activity and risks. Whereas measurements of height and weight have some useful meaning with regard to a person's general health, there is little if any significance to height and weight as important health criteria in the typical workplace. With respect to methodologies, preferred methods are not necessarily those that are most precise but, in some circumstances, may be those that can be performed most rapidly. Which tests to perform and which method to employ can only be decided by licensed medical authority—and these decisions must be made on a case-by-case basis.

The fact that decisions about the type of data and information required and the best means for obtaining that data and information are within the sole province of the physician does not mean that the safety officer has little or even no responsibility regarding the design of an effective and comprehensive medical surveillance program. On the contrary, it may be argued that no other responsibility of the safety officer is more demanding or requires more liaison and coordination with external medical authority. Of particular importance are the following considerations:

1. Most safety officers tend to assume that any licensed medical authority is suitable for the design and implementation of an in-plant medical surveillance program. This is definitely not the case. Where possible, the selection of medical professionals should be based on (a) professional experience in occupational medicine, (b) direct professional access to medical and analytical specialists and services regarding laboratory analyses and the timely processing of medically relevant data, and (c) demonstrated experience in quality control management of all professional services.

2. Even when contracting with medical professionals who have extensive experience in occupational medical specialties, the safety officer must understand the importance of providing these professionals with comprehensive baseline data and information on in-plant hazards. Such data and information includes not only facility-specific information on ambient concentrations of hazardous chemicals, but also all information regarding the potential health significance of those chemicals, such as the target organs of the chemicals themselves and of combustion products. While the safety officer might assume that medical professionals have this information, they often do not—which, given the tens of thousands of different chemicals in daily commerce, is understandable.

3. Despite the fact that the selection of appropriate medical testing of personnel is the professional responsibility of the medical professional, it is necessary that the corporate safety officer thoroughly understand the basis of selection, including (a) the range of different medical tests and procedures that can be performed, (b) alternative methods for performing the various tests and procedures, (c) interpretive criteria to be used in evaluating the significance of medical data and information, and (d) the limits associated with the use of any medical data or information for the purpose of diagnosing potential health conditions.

In this regard, the safety officer is well advised that, as with any contracted service affecting the health and safety of employees, any potential liability that might result from incompetence or oversight is not necessarily restricted to the contractor, but might also accrue to the company and corporate executives or managers. In short, it is always best to assume that the company is ultimately responsible for accepting and implementing the professional recommendations of its contractors, including the recommendations made by licensed medical authority.

4. Prior to committing to any professional medical surveillance service, the safety officer must ensure that medical surveillance reports will be presented in a format that provides for (a) ready comprehension of the significance of medical data and information by responsible corporate personnel and (b) professional documentation regarding any potential need for follow-up action or corporate response. Summaries of each type of health monitoring data (Figure 17.3) should clearly highlight the significance of findings and present the basis for the interpretation of that significance.

5. The processing and handling of any health-related information must be monitored assiduously to ensure confidentiality. The safety officer is strongly advised to examine in detail those control measures implemented by all relevant medical-service personnel (including external examining physicians and medical-testing laboratory personnel) and, where necessary, to demand additional safeguards.

Of particular importance is the need to ensure that physicians do not report any health information about employees to corporate personnel that does not directly relate to workplace conditions or fitness for assigned work. The reporting of medical monitoring results and the maintenance of medical records must be conducted in strict conformity with established rules governing confidentiality and should be closely coordinated with corporate legal counsel, corporate human resources personnel, and the legal counsel of medical contractors.

PROGRAMMATIC REVIEW

Once implemented, a medical surveillance program must be viewed as an essential lifeline for employees and should therefore be carefully monitored for effectiveness and efficiency. It is especially important that there be at least an annual review of the entire program, with particular care given to the following items:

1. A case-by-case review of any incident involving any aspect of the surveillance program, including episodic exposure to hazardous agents, medical monitoring data that required specific follow-up actions, and discernible trends in the frequency of episodic events or in monitoring data that may signify the need to review operational procedures or the use of personal protective equipment,

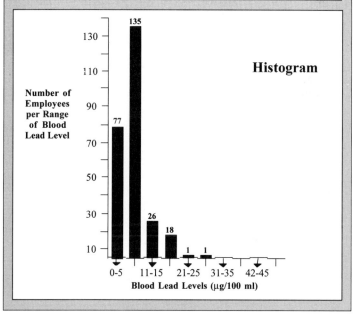

Blood Lead Levels

Inorganic lead is absorbed into the body through the lung and the intestinal tract. Organic lead can be absorbed through the lung, but the skin is the more common route.

In the studied population of workers, no overt signs of lead intoxication were identified in health history data or by means of the physical examination. The following histogram displays the distribution of the blood lead levels obtained in the 1990 survey of workers. No level met or exceeded the OSHA standard .

FIGURE 17.3   Example of a summary presentation of medical monitoring data regarding blood lead levels among industrial personnel. Such a concise verbal and graphic presentation of medical surveillance data is necessary in order to ensure that nonmedically trained corporate personnel understand the significance of detailed medical surveillance findings and the recommendations of physicians *(adapted from materials provided by Environmental Medicine Resources, Inc.).*

2. The need to include newly developed medical monitoring tests or to delete or modify other tests (e.g., frequency, methodology) in light of the state-of-art of industrial medical surveillance, changes in facility operations involving hazardous substances or conditions, in-plant ambient monitoring

data, or changes in regulatory requirements or applicable health and safety standards, and

3. Performance evaluation of medical service contractors, including attending physicians and analytical laboratories, with particular emphasis on (a) the timeliness, comprehensiveness, and clarity of written reports and recommendations, (b) adequacy of technical and scientific documentation, and (c) employee satisfaction.

It is recommended that, during this annual programmatic review, contracted medical personnel be requested to present an in-plant oral review of findings to date and discuss their own recommendations regarding any potential changes in the surveillance program.

CHAPTER 18

INTEGRATED PERSONNEL TRAINING

Personnel training requirements have become key requirements in regulations related to workplace health and safety. Their importance derives from two distinct although interrelated factors that have long influenced American workplace regulations: (a) the need for employees to develop the skills and behavioral patterns required to achieve and maintain safe work conditions and (b) the right of employees to participate in decision-making processes that affect their well being.

Given the diversity of health and safety regulations and the growing awareness of health and safety risks as well as alternative methods for controlling those risks, personnel training has become a complex undertaking for even small businesses and, in large corporations, often demands a significant investment of time and money. In both large and small corporations, the concept of "integrated personnel training" is increasingly relevant not only to broad health and safety objectives, but also to converging economic and marketing interests that underlie any modern business.

DIMENSIONS OF AN INTEGRATED TRAINING PROGRAM

Whatever the specific objectives of any type of training, all personnel training is today best viewed in the context of *corporate risk management*, which is inclusive of all corporate effort to control losses in productivity, capital resources, human resources, and market performance. Deficiencies in personnel training related to human health and safety, including not only the health and safety of employees but also of the public at large, must be assumed to contribute both directly and indirectly to such losses in terms of:

- direct health care costs for affected employees and public
- regulatory fines and other legal costs associated with civil and criminal proceedings related to environmental, health, and safety incidents
- insurance premiums that reflect the degree of health and safety risk containment
- facility audit costs associated with enforcement efforts of regulatory agencies
- remediation costs associated with the clean-up of contaminated sites
- loss of accreditation by national and international business and marketing associations, with consequent adverse impact on competitive standing within a global market
- loss of market share due to adverse publicity generated by health and safety incidents or conditions
- increased administrative costs due to incident reporting and follow-up, as well as recruitment and training of replacement personnel

In light of these considerations, it is clear that an in-plant health and safety training program must first be integrated with an overall business ethos that gives the highest priority to sound health, safety, and environmental (HSE) management practices—an ethos that, today, is rapidly becoming the essential managerial hallmark of any globally competitive enterprise and, consequently, a touchstone in modern graduate education programs in business management.

The fact that, more than 100 years after the advent of the industrial revolution, "the marketplace" has finally discovered the importance of human health and safety, should not diminish the key relevance of legally enforceable and technically complex regulations. Notwithstanding the persistent debate regarding the pros and cons of governmental intrusion into boardroom deliberation, the elevation of "good health and safety" practices to "good business" practices has occurred, in fact, only after regulatory agencies caught the serious attention of business.

The number of these regulations and the range of workplace standards they establish, whether attesting in political rhetoric to the demonstrable need of employees or, contrarily, simply to the overzealousness of bureaucrats, clearly define a range of potential workplace hazards to human health and safety that few if any would dare to refute before any objective audience. Setting the terms of a debate is sometimes even more important than resolving the details subject to debate.

With regard to workplace health and safety standards, OSHA has clearly circumscribed certain issues that must be addressed by personnel training regardless of potential future changes in regulatory strategy or philosophy, including:

1. Responsibility and accountability in the design and day-to-day management of the corporate health and safety program: Personnel training that does not clearly identify functional responsibilities and specific means for establishing and maintaining accountability for all policies, practices, and procedures regarding the safety of the workplace environment cannot be condoned under any circumstance and must be viewed as "prima facie" evidence that the corporation is primarily concerned with "paper compliance" with health and safety standards as opposed to the actual health and safety of its employees.

2. Behavioral measurements of the efficacy and adequacy of health and safety policies and procedures: The objective of any training must be objective-oriented communication, which is always a two-way flow of information between the trainer and the persons being trained. The one-way flow of information from an instructor or, as is more commonly the case, from video tapes, "canned" computerized programs, or pamphlets to a silent student is neither communication nor training. The only meaningful health and safety training is that which actually affects workplace behavior, and this can occur only when the training actively involves employees in relating discussed information to their specific workplace activities and responsibilities.

3. Active employee participation in all decision-making regarding health and safety: Effective personnel training must be based on the premise that health and safety is a joint objective and responsibility of both management and labor. Where health and safety practices and procedures (or the lack thereof) are perceived as emanating solely at the discretion of corporate management, it is unlikely that any personnel training program can have any measurable influence on workplace health or safety.

4. The importance of personnel training as a prerequisite to undertaking job assignment: Personnel training in health and safety practices and requirements is today an essential component of the initial in-plant processing of new employees. While it is neither possible nor desirable to attempt to complete all health and safety training prior to undertaking actual job assignments, the company must ensure that initial training is sufficient to ensure that workers are not at special health or safety risk simply because of their status as newly assigned personnel. This requires that the corporate health and safety training program be appropriately "tiered" or "staggered" to meet the needs of personnel at various stages of their employment, including the categories of newly hired, newly assigned, and temporary personnel, as well as personnel in need of refresher or advanced training, or additional training due to the implementation of new production processes or procedures.

TRAINING OBJECTIVES vs REGULATORY
COMPLIANCE OBJECTIVES

Regrettably, health and safety training objectives become confused with regulatory compliance objectives—a confusion that too often reflects a misguided corporate preoccupation with doing as little as possible to comply with specific regulations, which in turn, is an attitude that typically reflects an hierarchical isolation of upper level management from the realities of the modern workplace.

In the United States, for example, many executives would be surprised to learn that the Williams–Steiger Occupational Safety and Health Act of 1970, which is the congressional authority for OSHA, requires "that every employer covered under the Act furnish to his employees employment and a place of employment which are free from recognized hazards that are causing or are likely to cause death or serious physical harm to his employees (29 CFR 1903.1)." Thus, even in the absence of specific regulatory workplace standards (e.g., lockout/tagout, confined spaces, hazard communication, etc.), OSHA has the authority to act to protect the health and safety of workers.

In some jurisdictions, broad authority to ensure the health and safety of the citizen-worker is accomplished not only by legislative but also by constitutional means, as in India, where the Supreme Court in 1983 interpreted the constitutionally guaranteed right to life as requiring a healthy and safe environment, and in South Africa, where the newly elected democratic government included in its constitution the right of every citizen (including, it may be presumed, every worker) to an environment that is not detrimental to health and well-being. To these examples of the increasingly broad national and international mandate on behalf of human health and safety and environmental quality must be added the directives of the European Union, which are legally binding on its 12 member states and which, since 1973, have increasingly focused on the rights of citizens to a healthful and safe environment.

Where corporate executives understand that human health and safety and environmental quality are essential corporate objectives in an increasingly interactive global economy, it is well established that health and safety training of personnel must ensure regulatory compliance but must not be solely defined or constrained by or otherwise limited to specific regulatory requirements. In short, regulatory requirements are best viewed as *de minimus* requirements that apply under all circumstances. However, to ensure workplace health and safety, it is typically necessary to go well beyond published regulatory standards. To effectively integrate what may be required by written law and what is required by actual workplace circumstance to protect a worker is, accordingly, the fundamental objective of any health and safety training program.

TABLE 18.1   Example of Major Topics That Might Be Included in a Comprehensive Corporate
Training Policy Document Regarding Health and Safety Programs

---

Global Enterprises, Inc.

Training Policy
Health and Safety Programs

Table of Contents

1. Introduction
2. Programs and Responsibilities
3. Training Methods
4. Scheduling Constraints
5. Presenters
6. Training Records
7. General Policies
8. Specific Programmatic Requirements

Appendices

Appendix 1. Training Program Syllabus
Appendix 2. Training Attendance Form
Appendix 3. Employees Training
                   Evaluation Form
Appendix 4. Monitor's Training
                   Evaluation Form

TRAINING POLICY DOCUMENT

Historically, companies have devised separate training programs to meet the legal requirements of individual regulations regarding workplace health and safety, including specific requirements for personnel training. Given the increasing number of such regulations as well as the need (as discussed above) for health and safety training beyond *de minimus* regulatory requirements, corporations are well advised to develop a comprehensive policy document as a basic management tool for the design and implementation of all corporate health and safety training. Key elements of such a policy document are included in Table 18.1 and are summarized as follows:

Programs and Responsibilities

The objective of this section is to identify precisely the individual training programs that fall within the purview of this policy document and to assign specific responsibilities for the design, content, conduct, and quality management of each program. Programs to be included are (a) those required by regulations, such as "respiratory protection," "confined space and hot work permits," "bloodborne pathogens," etc., and (b) those deemed by corporate officials and employees as appropriate to workplace circumstances or otherwise desirable but not specifically addressed by existing workplace regulations, such as a training program on "general health and safety topics," "health and safety aspects of prescribed medicines," or "substance abuse."

Assigned responsibilities should include specific requirements regarding the review and revision of each program. Provision should also be made for the timely addition of new programs, including new topics and additional levels of training within the various programs.

Training Methods

For each training program, specific training methods should be identified on the basis of which method or combination of methods is most likely to achieve behavioral and informational objectives. Regardless of personal preferences, a comprehensive range of methods should be evaluated for efficacy, including (but not limited to) the following:

- classroom style lectures
- demonstrations
- roundtable workshops or problem solving sessions
- seminars
- audio-visual programs
- topical discussions
- on-the-job practicums
- table-top and "field" exercises
- site visits to other facilities

While on-the-job training is a valuable approach, it must be emphasized that on-the-job training must be carefully evaluated in regard to (a) relevant regulatory requirements and (b) the risk to which the person being trained will be exposed. Generally, on-the-job training should be considered only when initial training has been completed in a context that does not involve undue hazard or risk.

Scheduling Constraints

Training schedules that are determined solely by routine work schedules are typically irrelevant to training objectives. The time required for a particular training session is precisely the time required to achieve specifically stated and monitored behavioral and informational objectives and should not be determined by any other factor. For example, while it may be convenient to train employees at the end of an 8-hr shift, it is hardly surprising that such training is frequently a waste of time and effort. The schedule for training in each program should be established to ensure the most meaningful involvement of employees with the training exercise—an objective that can be met only by considering the type of information to be discussed, the nature of the exercise, and the mental and physical condition of the workers to be trained.

Presenters

While many companies have tended to utilize consultants as trainers, the range of health and safety training is today sufficiently broad that both in-house personnel as well as consultants should be considered for the presentation of training programs. The actual selection, of course, depends upon the type of information to be discussed and the relevance of the presenter's credentials to that type of information. In some instances, priority must be given to academic or professional credentials; in some, to practical experience. The types and balance of the presenter's academic, professional, and experiential credentials should be specified for each training program, as well as those personal skills and attributes that are considered essential for the achievement of specific training objectives. All presenters of personnel training programs should provide the company with a detailed resume of relevant experience as well as a syllabus for the program and a copy of any training materials used during the presentation. It is recommended that the corporation always reserve the right to make an audio or audio-visual recording of any health and safety training program presented by either in-house personnel or consultants, as well as the right to use any recording for purposes of documentation, quality control, and/or for subsequent training purposes.

Training Records

In addition to the documents provided by each presenter (i.e., resume, syllabus, and course materials), the safety officer should maintain the following documents for each training session:

- Training attendance form: to include the name of the program, the name of the presenter, the date of presentation, and the printed name and signatures of training participants

- Employee's training evaluation form: to be submitted by each program participant upon completion of the training and to include a detailed assessment of the content of the training, the quality of the presentation, and the usefulness of the training
- Monitor's training evaluation form: to be completed by a designated company employee who attends the training for the express purpose of evaluating the content and presentation of the training

The increasing use of training evaluation forms, whether completed by training participants or by specially designated monitors, requires appropriate documentation regarding actions subsequently taken in response to those evaluations, including any revision of training session contents and the replacement of presenters. At least an annual review of all training evaluations should be conducted, with appropriate documentation of findings and consequent actions.

Additional documents may also be required, such as the results of written examinations or exercises that many companies increasingly use to measure and document the efficacy of in-house training. In some instances, companies also include post-training evaluation forms that document the assessment of workplace behavior of individuals who have completed various stages of training. Documentation of "personnel actions" undertaken by a human resource department due to inappropriate employee behavior or activity specifically addressed in previous health and safety training is also often included as part of the documentation associated with that training.

General Policies

This section is devoted to those policies that must guide and inform the overall training effort, such as:

- assessment of efficacy of training
- programmatic review and revision
- availability of resource information on health and safety issues
- relationship between workplace health and safety and general lifestyle
- employee participation in health and safety decision-making
- state-of-the-art standards and procedures

In developing these policies, the company must understand that they are increasingly subject to external legal scrutiny, especially with regard to the correspondence between written policies and the manner in which they are actually executed (or ignored) in the workplace. The basic rule to follow is that adage: "Say what you mean, and mean what you say."

Specific Programmatic Requirements

In this section, all requirements for each health and safety program are collated, with particular emphasis given to the following items:

- Regulatory reference for program (e.g., "respiratory protection")
- Behavioral and informational objectives
- Personnel to be trained (by job categories and work status, as in "new employees," "office personnel," "temporary laboratory personnel," etc.)
- Frequency of presentation
- Method of evaluation of effectiveness
- Responsibility for design, implementation, review, and revision

SPECIAL CONCERNS

Regardless of the size of a company, the management of personnel training related to health and safety demands an important investment of time and effort which, though arguably a necessary insurance against regulatory, criminal, and civil law proceedings, is at risk of numerous factors that can easily overcome the best of intent.

Some of these stubbornly difficult factors are directly related to the simple fact that the act of training is inextricably connected to the act of learning. While the failure to train is very often the failure to learn, in matters related to workplace health and safety it is the corporation's responsibility to train that receives primary attention—with the consequence that an employee who refuses to learn or to change workplace behavior in accordance with good health and safety practices and who thereby suffers an injury is likely to benefit economically at the expense of the company.

It is therefore clearly incumbent upon a company not only to devise clearly competent training programs, but also to implement stringent personnel actions whenever employees who have completed that training nonetheless fail to translate training lessons into workplace behavior. Yet, even then the company is typically constrained by a wide range of legal and societal standards that may often serve to protect a worker from the consequences of his own intransigence or incompetence.

Certainly one can empathize with a business manager who, unlike a teacher in a college or university, is typically to be blamed for the failure of someone else to learn. However, that same manager should understand that empathy is not necessarily the guarantor of sympathy. The fact remains that, in the modern world, a business does have the responsibility to make every reasonable effort to inform and instruct its employees as to the proper means for working safely—and, by proper monitoring of personnel, to ensure they translate training into appropriate workplace behavior. Regardless of the attendant difficulties and frustrations, health and safety training and all that it implies is a basic cost of doing business. In light of the clearly dismal history of worker health and safety throughout most of the industrial revolution, one might reasonably add, "Finally!"

In undertaking its admittedly burdensome and difficult task of translating training into safe workplace behavior, any business must come to grips with two key issues that, regardless of a company's size or geographic location or industrial code, typically demand particular attention.

Professional Managerial Skills

The overall responsibility for personnel training in health and safety matters is most often given to a safety or training officer or other persons who, regardless of the extent of their technical, scientific, or other skills, are not professionally trained managers. What managerial skills they do possess have typically been obtained through limited on-the-job experience, with little if any guidance or instruction by professional managers. Perceived as essentially technicians, they occupy relatively low-level and low-status positions in a corporate hierarchy that, minimizing their authority even while expanding their responsibility, effectively defines their contribution as a white-collar service function that, at best, is seen as subservient to both mainline corporate managerial and production tasks.

While more sophisticated corporations have in recent years begun to elevate the status of personnel training by assigning this function to higher level departments, such as a human resource or loss control department, or even, in very few cases, to executive level officers, the vast majority of companies persist in marginalizing personnel training. The consequence is that the typical safety or training officer is essentially ignorant of basic managerial skills, especially those related to the management of information, quality control, and objective-oriented systems analysis.

Consider the fact, for example, that even a small manufacturing company having on the order of 40 employees may be legally required to comply with a dozen or more relatively complex health and safety regulations—including, for example, lockout/tagout, confined space and hot work, respiratory protection, management of change, bloodborne pathogens, spill control and emergency response, electrical safety, hazard communication, laboratory safety, hearing conservation, etc.

In addition to these regulations, each of which specifically requires health and safety training of personnel, the same company may have a variety of additional health and safety training requirements imposed by the concerns of corporate executives, insurance carriers, corporate owners, unions, and the general public. In this rather common situation, which specific employees must be trained in what, to what degree or level of competence, how often, and with what measure of success or failure are rather fundamental questions—and yet, few safety officers who have mainline training responsibility can immediately provide the answers or even know how to organize a relevant data base or computerize a data base to generate the answers.

The prevailing ignorance of safety officers with respect to basic managerial skills, and the consequent ineffectiveness of much of the health and training programs conducted within corporations cannot be blamed on the safety officer but, rather, should be attributed to that corporate executive who considers the management of finances, productivity, raw materials, and product distribution to be inestimably more important than the management of human health and safety—that corporate executive who, despite a long reign in the history of corporations, is well poised to become an endangered species throughout the world.

The Realities of Communication

That there can be no effective training without effective communication is a bromide so logically soporific it is usually ignored in practice, especially in the United States where the Americanized English language is considered the *lingua franca* that not only overcomes all linguistic and cultural barriers but also obviates any and all distinctions imposed by diverse personal experience and values.

The perception is, of course, quite wrong—as evidenced in the United States by the rapidly expanding influx of non-English speaking persons into the work force as well as by the tardy and painful recognition that many of our English-speaking fellow citizens, including some with college degrees, are in fact functionally illiterate.

The political rhetoric that bemoans this real situation and that would implement a "suitably patriotic" solution, as well as regulatory requirements regarding the use of English in warning signs and labels are, however, absolutely irrelevant to the fact that, for now and for the foreseeable future, corporate health and safety training must effectively confront the linguistic pluralism of the American workforce whether that pluralism derives from differences in primary language, from differences in language skills or, for that matter, from differences in linguistic expression and cognition imposed by personal and social experience. To do otherwise is essentially equivalent to defining worker health and safety as a reward of social conformity rather than as a right regardless of human diversity.

   The enormous difficulty inherent in the act of communication within an actual linguistic, cultural, and experiential pluralism cannot be made any the less, of course, simply by extolling the importance of the common objective of human health and safety—nor is the American experiment in linguistic diversity yet so far progressed as to give universally relevant clues as to the most effective strategies for dealing with that difficulty. However, we do know that one does not overcome it simply by speaking English more loudly and more slowly! We also know that the American business community, which is increasingly dependent for its very livelihood upon communication across cultural and linguistic barriers, has had to begin to divest itself of its traditional linguistic and cultural isolationism and to experiment with practical means of fostering cross-cultural and linguistic fluency. Finally, we know that computer technology has only begun to be tapped for its contribution to human communication whether in the university, at home, or in business. With a realistic understanding of the limitations of any language, with an experimental approach toward achieving business objectives despite those limitations, and with a sophisticated electronic technology simply waiting to be used, we already perceive that perhaps our standard approach to education and training is already grossly outdated and in need of new and as yet untested approaches.

CHAPTER 19

DATA AND INFORMATION
MANAGEMENT

A sufficient health and safety program is data- and information-intensive—not only in terms of the level of detail, but also in terms of the diversity of data and information that must be considered. The management of that data and information is therefore absolutely critical to the success of a health and safety program and, as emphasized in Chapters 1 and 20, to both short- and long-term business objectives.

Given the widespread accessibility to global informational networks and the ready availability of an ever-expanding computer technology, it might appear that the management of health and safety data and information should be a relatively simple task. However, it is well worth considering that access to global data banks and informational networks enhances not only the potential for improvement in the efficiency and comprehensiveness of decision-making but also the potential for utter confusion. Even the most sophisticated technology for retrieving and processing information is absolutely no guarantor of competence, nor can it correct the consequences of incompetence.

COMMON MISCONCEPTIONS

As happens with the application of any new technology, the application of computer technology to the needs defined by a comprehensive workplace health and safety program is subject to a variety of misconceptions that can actually contravene the objectives of that program. Some of the most common misconceptions that should receive careful consideration by the safety officer are as follows:

A Tool—Not a Guru

Despite the continuing development of so-called "expert programs," computers are essentially tools. While an extremely powerful tool in terms of flexibility, efficiency, and range of application, a computer cannot as yet even begin to substitute for human intelligence. The practical consequence of this simple fact for the safety officer must be the realization that any aspect of a health and safety program must be fully conceived and developed before appropriate computerization may be attempted—and even then, only when the specific objectives of computerization can be clearly defined in terms of the needs of the program.

The Prevalence of Bad Information

The rapidity with which we can now access worldwide data bases means that we can as quickly retrieve bad information as we can good information. In fact, one may reasonably suppose that the likelihood of retrieving bad information, pure nonsense, or at least misleading data is far greater than retrieving information that is subject to strict quality criteria and review. The practical consequence of this situation for the safety officer must be the realization that data and information to be included in a health and safety program must be evaluated for its veracity and pertinence regardless of source.

Follow the Program or Program the Objective

Software marketing hoopla to the contrary, there is no single computer program that can meet all the needs of a comprehensive health and safety program. Each program has its capacities and its limitations—and both its capacities and its limitations are inherently obstinate. The practical consequence of this for the safety officer must be the realization that the capacities and limitations of each program must be carefully evaluated with regard to the objectives of the health and safety program. There is, in short, no such thing as "an excellent program" except that it meets precisely defined needs.

Given the importance that a computer program serve the needs of health and safety objectives and not *vice versa*, the safety officer should consider the wisdom of developing custom-made computer programming rather than relying upon commercially available "canned" programs. While this alternative is typically given little serious attention by those having responsibility for in-plant health and safety, it should be noted that few companies entrust their financial or inventory or billing procedures to "over the counter" computer programs but, rather, utilize the consulting services of professional programmers.

The Gospel by Geek

In many companies having extensively computerized operations, and especially where such operations entail the use of mainframe computers, computer programs and procedures are typically centralized in a computer operations or data processing department. Even where PC networking as opposed to mainframe systems are employed, such a centralized department usually exerts full authority over all computer hardware and software. Certainly there are very good reasons for this, including the need for data and information security and the "handshaking" requirements of computer networks.

However, it is reasonable to suggest that there are practical levels of flexibility required in order to ensure that the needs of corporate financial management, inventory control, and office management do not unnecessarily constrain the operational needs of the health and safety program. In proposing appropriate computerization of the various elements of a health and safety program, the safety officer must therefore define capabilities that may be peculiar to health and safety management and that should not be restricted by the algorithms of other computer-assisted corporate functions and operations.

Of particular importance is the need to conduct at least an annual review of the efficacy of any computer-assisted aspects of a health and safety program—a review that should not in any manner be constrained by otherwise overriding corporate computer-related operations or policies.

ELEMENTS OF THE IN-PLANT DATA AND INFORMATION BASE

While the data and information base for a health and safety program must be site-specific, there are certain types of data and information that have a universal relevance. Examples of minimal types of data and information bases and necessary cross-referencing among individual data bases may be briefly summarized as follows:

1. Persons at potential risk:

   - corporate personnel by name and job category, with cross-reference to source of potential risk or hazard, pertinent regulations, training needs, required protective equipment, required medical surveillance, and personal susceptibilities or other factors of special relevance to health and safety

- other on-site persons, including visitors, contractors, consultants, and vendors, with cross-reference to specific health and safety precautions, restrictions, and other corporate policies and procedures regarding health and safety
- off-site persons who may be exposed to hazards associated with plant operations, including property abutters, downwind or downstream residents and communities, with cross-reference to environmental mechanisms of dispersal of hazardous materials and substances, automatic and manual alarm devices and systems, and corporate emergency procedures and requirements
- on-site emergency responders, including corporate personnel and community-based responders, with cross-reference to equipment and communication needs, decontamination and waste disposal requirements, first aid and medical treatment requirements, and other relevant corporate policies and procedures

2. Inventory and evaluation of hazards:

- Types of physical, chemical, or biological hazards, with cross-reference to source, modes of exposure, chronic and acute effects, signs and symptoms of exposure, emergency and follow-up treatment, or medical surveillance
- Sources of routine and emergency hazards, with cross-reference to required engineering and managerial controls, required use of personal protective equipment, routine and emergency ambient monitoring requirements, inspection schedules, and evaluation criteria

3. Incident response:

- Description of individual health and safety incidents (including routine and emergency incidents), with detailed assessment of cause and cross-reference to pertinent regulatory requirements, corporate policies, and specific requirements of the health and safety program
- Assessment of frequency of magnitude of incidents, with cross-reference to review and modification of the health and safety program, notification of regulatory authorities, and personnel training requirements

4. Reference resources:

- Consultant, contractor, regulatory, and other available personnel having special knowledge and experience relevant to health and safety, with cross-reference to specific data and informational needs of the corporate health and safety program

- Hardcopy and electronic sources of regulatory, technical, and scientific data and information, with cross-reference to routine and emergency need for information, including up-to-date information on health and safety standards, chemical toxicity and compatibility, personal protective equipment, monitoring devices, and medical treatment and surveillance
- In-place maps, schematics, and diagrams for all plant structures and properties that locate all primary sources of hazards, routes of ingress and egress, potential pathways and receiving systems for accidental spills or releases of hazardous materials, with cross-reference to specific regulatory requirements (e.g., underground storage tanks, hazardous waste storage areas, electrical transformers) and the requirements of specific corporate health and safety programs

It must be stressed that the above types of data and information should be immediately available to the safety officer whether or not the data and information are computerized. However, the cross-referencing required to meet the pressing needs of an in-plant emergency, a facility inspection by regulatory personnel, or even routine operational decision-making clearly emphasizes the importance of well designed and highly integrated computerized files.

EXTERNAL DATA BASES

Electronic publishing is a rapidly expanding phenomenon that commercial companies, professional organizations, and governmental agencies increasingly use to make technical and scientific information and data more easily available to the safety officer at little to moderate cost. Powerful "search and retrieve" programs, CD ROMs, and worldwide networking provide essentially instantaneous access to data and information on all aspects of workplace health and safety, including state, national, and international regulations, health and safety standards, epidemiological and laboratory studies, protective clothing and equipment, and ambient and personal monitoring systems.

While it is important that the safety officer explore the full range of available data bases, it is equally important that the safety officer keep very much in mind the following guidelines:

1. Even a brief perusal of health and safety standards is sufficient to determine that standards are highly variable from one legal jurisdiction to another. While it goes without saying that the safety officer must ensure compliance with the specific legal authority having jurisdiction over his or

her company, it may very well be appropriate to adopt a more stringent standard proposed by some other authority. Such an approach is consistent with not only the principle of minimizing health and safety risk, but also the recognition that there is often a significant lag between scientific findings and regulatory reform. Of course, there are instances in which standards become less stringent precisely because of advances in scientific understanding of hazards and risks—a consideration that should nonetheless be weighed against the industrial state-of-the-art.

2. There are many CD ROM data bases on chemical hazards and risks, some of which are available through chemical manufacturers and some through commercial sources, including companies that specialize in the production of material safety data sheets (MSDSs). A comparison of MSDSs prepared by different companies for the same chemical substance or product will often reveal differences regarding not only specific hazards, but also routes of entry, target organs, and recommended protective clothing and equipment.

The safety officer must understand that the adoption of the findings, determinations, and recommendations made by any purveyor of information does not absolve the buyer or user of such information from potential liabilities that might accrue to errors of fact or judgment on which that information is based. It is therefore necessary that comparisons of alternative data bases be examined and, where differences do occur, that the safety officer assume the responsibility for resolving discrepancies.

In many instances, discrepancies in hazard determinations and the toxicology of chemicals are not due to oversight or error, but to differences in the interpretation of highly technical data. Where this is the case, the safety officer must seek guidance from both regulatory and competent scientific authority and not simply accept the judgment as presented in a particular data base.

3. While many commercial electronic data bases are offered as part of a subscription service, which ensures periodic updating of information, the safety officer must have confidence that data bases used for day-to-day decision-making regarding human health and safety are, in fact, current and represent the best available understanding in industrial hygiene and hazard management.

Such confidence is warranted only where the safety officer is able to commit resources for the express purpose of reviewing data bases and testing their content against recognized legal, professional, and scientific standards. For example, it is strongly recommended that, at least annually, the safety officer carefully review recent governmental reports related to workplace health and safety that are readily available through the National Technical Information Service (NTIS) of the Technology Administration in the U.S. Department of Commerce (telnet via Internet: fedworld.gov; telnet via World

Wide Web Services: URL http://www.fedworld.gov). Of course, other sources should also be considered, including such sources as the National Fire Protection Association (NFPA), National Institute of Occupational Safety and Health (NIOSH), Occupational Safety and Health Administration (OSHA), and the Agency for Toxic Substances and Disease Registry of the U.S. Public Health Service (USPHS).

INTERNAL DATA BASES

As important as external data bases are, they cannot substitute for those data bases that must be compiled on a site-specific basis and which represent the operational details of any corporate health and safety plan. Encompassing all corporate health and safety policies and procedures regarding potential site hazards, engineering and operational controls, personnel risk factors, ambient monitoring, medical surveillance, facility auditing and inspection, and personnel training, internal data bases must not only accommodate the documentation needs of the health and safety program, but also meet the day-to-day operational needs of that program, including:

- scheduling of key activities (e.g., ambient monitoring, personnel training, medical surveillance, internal audits of operations)
- assessment of health and safety incidents
- revision of pertinent programs and policies in light of in-plant incidents, changes in health and safety standards, changes in facility operations, or changes in regulatory requirements
- personnel actions required to enforce health and safety policies and procedures
- assessment of effectiveness of engineering and operational controls of hazards as well as of personal protective equipment
- evaluation of in-place policies and procedures with regard to the current and developing state-of-art
- periodic assessment of potential health and safety effects of plant operations on the surrounding community, including both routine and emergency operations

In constructing internal data bases, which includes the incorporation of selected data and information obtained from external sources, the safety officer is well advised to focus on specific information that is most likely to be immediately needed under foreseeable circumstances. For example, what information will be immediately required:

- in case of a fire emergency—by community fire fighting personnel, by internal emergency response personnel, by other community services?

- for the purpose of an internal corporate review of on-site engineering control measures regarding the accidental spill of bulk hazardous liquids?
- in a situation involving employee symptoms of possible chemical exposure?

Only by defining the particular informational needs engendered by circumstances such as these can the safety officer begin to identify specific cross-reference capabilities of the diverse data bases necessarily included in a comprehensive health and safety program—capabilities that ultimately determine the actual usefulness of those data bases and which, unfortunately, are too often overlooked by personnel so enraptured by the sheer volume of information at their command that they forget that no information is of any value whatsoever unless it can be efficiently integrated with specific objectives.

TEAM APPROACH

It is strongly recommended that the safety officer not attempt to construct a data base except through the joint effort of a team composed of personnel who, by virtue of their workplace responsibility, authority, and experience, reflect the range of potential informational needs that can be directly associated with a health and safety data base. Ideally, such a team would consist of higher level corporate executive personnel, legal counsel, managerial and supervisory personnel, and other personnel having specific responsibility for internal health and safety programs and policies and for liaison with community authorities.

Such a broadly based team is necessary in order to ensure that the health and safety data base is comprehensively integrated with the needs of corporate planning and financing, operations management, human resource management, and environmental quality management. Corporate planning, after all, must be conducted with full awareness of employee and community risks associated with product development; financial decisions must be informed by potential needs regarding engineering and operational controls of both on-site and off-site hazards; short- and long-term operational schedules must take due account of health and safety requirements and procedures; human resource management must be tightly coupled to health and safety policies and objectives; and broad environmental objectives must be reflected in and entirely consistent with all aspects of workplace health and safety.

Once the team has developed its preliminary recommendations regarding the structure and contents of a health and safety data base, external authorities should be given the opportunity to review and comment upon those capabilities of the data management system that directly pertain to their responsibilities. Such authorities should include, at a minimum, the local fire chief, the coordinator of community services related to emergencies involving hazardous materials and chemicals, and local medical authorities who must respond to both in-plant and communitywide emergencies. Such authorities may have specific informational needs, either in substance or format, that should be incorporated into the corporate health and safety data base (e.g., information regarding the atmospheric dispersal of potentially fugitive chemical vapors, hardware and software compatibility between corporate data bases and mobile data processing units increasingly employed by emergency response personnel).

It should be noted that, in addition to these practical benefits, employing such a team approach to devising an in-plant health and safety data base also clearly reflects a fact that cannot be overemphasized—that a comprehensive and effective health and safety program is a corporatewide responsibility and a joint corporate and community commitment.

TABLE-TOP EXERCISES

Table-top exercises are discussed in Chapter 13 in terms of their use as a quality control measure of emergency preparedness. The safety officer should also give serious consideration to the use of table-top exercises for the purpose of testing the adequacy of health and safety data bases and management systems. This can be done in conjunction with training sessions on emergency preparedness or solely for the purpose of assessing the adequacy of data and information management systems.

A very practical approach to such an assessment is to define a variety of scenarios (e.g., accidental spill of bulk hazardous liquid) that would, if they actually occurred, require immediate access to particular types of information. In such an exercise, the objective is not simply to retrieve the appropriate information but, rather, to test the range of factors that may influence the successful retrieval and subsequent processing or use of the retrieved information. Of particular concern should be such considerations as follows:

1. How does the on-site person faced with a particular problem determine which information in the data base is required or at least most relevant?

2. Can the information be retrieved by persons most likely to be available at the time required, or must it be retrieved by a limited number of personnel who may not be available in a timely fashion?

3. How can the data required for a critical situation be retrieved or processed in the case of a power failure? Are printed records containing the needed information readily available under emergency conditions?

4. Does the retrieved information direct the person who retrieves it as to how to act upon it—or is it simply assumed that available personnel will know what to do with the information?

As attested by such questions, the overriding concern that must guide the construction of any extensive data base and data management system is that no single datum or bit of information can "speak for itself." What information do I need? How do I get it? What do I do with it? These are the necessary previous questions to any data management system and they cannot as yet be obviated by our most sophisticated electronic tools. Unasked or unanswered, clearly and precisely, they transform the most extensive data base into simply so many gigabits of nonsense.

CHAPTER 20

BUSINESS MANAGEMENT, HEALTH AND SAFETY, AND ENVIRONMENTAL QUALITY: AN ASSESSMENT OF TRENDS

Over the past 20 years in the United States, environmental as well as occupational health and safety regulations have given a progressive emphasis to the identification of personnel having specific responsibilities for the design, implementation, and day-to-day management of regulatory compliance programs. This focus on assigned responsibility is reflected in such regulatory terms as "chemical hygiene officer," "hazardous waste manager," "emergency response coordinator," "authorized personnel," and "right-to-know coordinator"—terms that, while not typically included in the historical categories of industrial job descriptions, define legally required tasks and job responsibilities to be associated with those descriptions.

The relatively rapid expansion of specific responsibilities associated with corporate compliance with environmental and occupational health and safety regulations and the essentially *ad hoc* assignment of these responsibilities in a context of traditional corporate departments and functions frequently result in substantial confusion regarding the practical workplace balance of personal responsibility and authority—a situation that is already a significant stimulus for reevaluating the relevance of traditional bureaucratic structures to ensure regulatory compliance by the modern corporation.

AUTHORITY vs RESPONSIBILITY

At the heart of any bureaucracy, whether explicitly stated or, as most often the case, only to be inferred from organizational structure, is the distinction between authority and responsibility—the first being, in essence, the right to exact the obedience of others while exercising the prerogatives of independent determination and judgment; the latter, the duty or obligation to be met through the exercise of that authority. One implies the other and, in consequence, the concepts of authority and responsibility become intimately interconnected in both the enculturated expectations of everyday life and the more formal principles and doctrines that guide institutional behavior.

However, of course, the marvel of all cultural traditions is that they are often easily "short-circuited"—modified to meet the demands of new experience or, as may often be the case, simply ignored. With regard to corporate attitudes toward environmental quality and human health, it would appear that the traditional sense of the need for a commensurate balance between authority and responsibility has much more frequently been purposely ignored than usefully modified.

Despite a growing number of exceptions, the corporate employee who is assigned programmatic environmental or health and safety responsibility is typically a low-level manager, supervisor, or technician who has little if any discernible authority over—or measurable influence on—key corporate decision-making or over any substantive planning or production-related process. In such a situation, it is not surprising that the safety officer usually becomes preoccupied with actual health and safety incidents and regulatory compliance failures rather than effectively managing a comprehensive health and safety program—or that the workplace continues to be the focus of governmental and social concern about human health and environmental quality.

The only practical way by which to ensure that the authority of corporate safety officials is in fact commensurate with their responsibility is to extend that authority to whatever extent required for the effective managerial control of the sources of health and safety hazards and of all circumstances that may contribute to or be affected by human exposure to those hazards. State-of-the-art companies today understand that this approach requires that health and safety responsibility be matched with high level executive authority—a recognition reflected in the fact that a growing number of graduate programs in business schools include curricula devoted to environmental quality and human health issues.

PROACTIVE vs REACTIVE MANAGEMENT

The traditional western business philosophy has largely emphasized the importance of responding to critical problems that develop in the manufacturing process, in marketing, in product development, and, perhaps less frequently but certainly with equal vigor, in the procurement of raw materials, in financial markets, and in the availability of suitable labor. Historically, this emphasis on reactive corporate capability has been entirely consistent with a persistent business ethos that demands rapid return on investment—an ethos that, being *now* oriented, concentrates corporate problem-solving efforts on clear and present problems that, if left unresolved, would endanger rapid financial return on investment. Such a philosophy has little if any regard for possible problems and generally relegates any serious concern about future "what ifs" to the impractical musings of idle (and most probably quite incompetent) minds.

With the rapid development of governmental regulations related to environmental quality and workplace health and safety and, perhaps even more importantly, the explosion of case law involving so-called "toxic torts," the practical effectiveness of this traditional business ethos has become rudely challenged by the realization that, not only are the financial profits on business investment at dire risk of a company's mismanagement of human health and the environment, but such mismanagement may well actually increase the liability of investors rather than, as for so long so devoutly believed by so many investors, minimize that liability.

A good example of the profound limitations of a reactive as opposed to a proactive approach to the corporate management of health risks and financial liability is afforded by alternative approaches to the management of reproductive risks in the workplace. For example, where production process chemicals are known to be either teratogenic or mutagenic, a company may consider that the most direct way of dealing with "the problem" is simply to allow work involving those chemicals to be performed only by those employees who are willing to sign a waiver that supposedly holds the company blameless for any abnormal fetus.

However, it is not at all clear that such a waiver will withstand legal scrutiny—especially in regard to the seminal legal question as to whether or not any employee may sign away what many consider to be legal human rights to a healthful environment. Moreover, such a waiver cannot in any way protect a company against a later suit initiated not by the employee whose fetus was injured but by the claimant who was that fetus. Finally, such a quick fix does not even begin to address the real issue, which is how best to reduce health risk to as low a level as possible.

The proactive approach in such a situation begins at defining the problem not in terms of the ultimate effect of a chemical exposure (i.e., an abnormal fetus) but, rather, in terms of the exposure itself—an issue that can and should be evaluated well before the adoption of a production-related chemical process that involves such hazardous chemicals. Proactively, one facet of the newly defined problem may require the company to implement a policy of reviewing all feedstock chemicals for the purpose of using, where possible, chemical substitutes that obviate or at least minimize reproductive risks. Another may require an in-depth analysis of state-of-the-art handling and ambient monitoring of those hazardous chemicals for which there are no less hazardous substitutes; still another may underscore the importance of specialized training for potentially exposed employees as well as alternative medical surveillance techniques.

MUTUAL vs COMPETITIVE INTERESTS

Both the popular and specialized literature on organizational behavior is replete with the seemingly infinitely diverse methods and absolutely imaginative means whereby individuals and groups methodically accrue to themselves the physical, economic, social, and psychological spoils of that most persistent of human pastimes, competition. To speak of the management of health and safety in the workplace without recognizing that any health and safety program must exist within a context of actively contending competitive interests would be totally unrealistic. Investments of personnel time and money to ensure state-of-the-art spill control capability imply (or at least may be perceived to imply) less time and money available for updating data processing, or replacing an outmoded cafeteria, or constructing a new operations building. Personnel training requirements for health and safety objectives may conflict (or at least may be perceived to conflict) with targeted productivity rates. Operational constraints imposed by a safety officer may infringe upon (or at least may be perceived to infringe upon) the traditional responsibilities and authority (and therefore the traditional status) of a shift foreman or a production manager.

As a general rule, any change introduced into an existing bureaucracy must be expected to trigger the proverbial turf battle that, if overlooked or ignored by management, usually evolves rapidly into an outright war in which there are few if any prohibited weapons. As a relatively new addition to the long tested structural hierarchies of business enterprise, health and safety personnel and programs are therefore vulnerable to the mayhem—and particularly so when upper level executive officers fail to emphasize that, as a matter of corporate policy, health and safety objectives as well as environmental quality objectives are in fact necessarily intrinsic to all other objectives—that environmental quality and human health and safety define the basic context in which all other business objectives are to be pursued, and that all corporate employees will be held responsible for the effective and efficient integration of health, safety, and environmental policies with all workplace activities.

REGULATORY CONSIDERATIONS

The relationship of authority and responsibility, proactive and reactive tendencies, and mutual and competitive interests, which are perennial internal concerns in any corporation under any circumstance, must also be directly influenced by regulatory philosophies and strategies imposed by the external world. It is therefore important to consider certain regulatory trends that are clearly discernible over the past 20 years and which promise to become even more clearly defined.

While some of the more recent approaches to the effective management of environmental quality and workplace health and safety have emphasized economic incentives, the basic approach has most frequently been the so-called "command and control" or regulatory approach. Despite a continuing interest in the potential for using market and other economic incentives to achieve health, safety, and environmental goals, the general consensus is (although sometimes grudgingly granted) that environmental objectives cannot be achieved in the absence of strict enforcement of clearly stated design and performance standards. In the United States, the setting and enforcement of such standards occurs at the Federal, state, and even local levels.

The basic American reliance on statutory law does not, of course, preclude the use of other legal mechanisms, including common law (or, in the case of Louisiana, Roman law), criminal law, and formal equity proceedings. In fact, some American statutes actually achieve their primary enforcement rigor by facilitating alternative forms of legal redress. This is usually achieved through the doctrine of "full disclosure."

For example, the Hazard Communication Standard (29 CFR 1910.1200; Chapter 5) requires employers to identify the hazards of all chemicals present at the work place and to train employees both in the types of hazards that may be encountered and the proper means of ensuring their protection. While statutory enforcement essentially relies upon an inspection of the written documentation associated with this standard, perhaps the most important factor influencing actual compliance is the threat of common law suits by employees who, having learned in some detail of the possible health effects of workplace chemicals, are increasingly prone to relate the state of their health to workplace conditions.

It is worth emphasizing three aspects of this standard—aspects that apply equally to other environmental and health and safety regulations.

First, it is clear that no Federal or state regulatory agency can ever employ sufficient enforcement personnel to inspect each and every workplace with any reasonable frequency. An obviously practical alternative, then, is to transform the employer's own employees into inspectors.

Second, in place of fines to be paid to an agency, which—despite ever increasing amounts—are generally limited, the effective inflation of the price of noncompliance to a common law compensatory and (most likely) punitive award substantially raises the stakes of noncompliance.

Third, once a common law suit is initiated, it is highly unlikely that the financial risk will be restricted to the corporation; more likely, the personal financial assets of owners, the chief executive officer, and other high level corporate officials and managers will also be at risk.

In a society such as the United States, whose public holds lawyers in almost as low esteem as governmental officials, these three eminently practical consequences of full disclosure are often derided as simply "job security for lawyers"—a conclusion that is potentially politically important in light of the fact that over 90% of federal funds devoted to the clean-up of hazardous waste sites has in fact been spent on lawyers' fees rather than actual clean-up operations.

On the other hand, it may also be argued that, regardless of the monetary cost, the increase in litigation engendered by full disclosure is a small price to pay for achieving environmental objectives that the American public has consistently supported over essentially the last full generation. Moreover, it might also be suggested that even substantial increases in litigation must be viewed in the context of an evolving history—i.e., from a period (which is still the present) in which the threat of exorbitant litigative awards and fees must be exercised in order to establish a new workplace ethic that, in the future, will not require such costly oversight control.

Other regulations regarding workplace health and safety also make use of full disclosure as part of a *de facto* compliance strategy. For example, regulations regarding energy management (29 CFR 1910.147; Chapter 7), confined spaces (29 CFR 1910.146; Chapter 8), and respiratory protection (29 CFR 1910.134; Chapter 10) require the development of written plans for achieving regulatory objectives. These plans, which effectively serve as contracts between the corporation, its employees, and OSHA, must be available for inspection not only by OSHA but also by employees. Employees must, in fact, receive specific training in the contents of such plans.

Still another American statute (Superfund Amendments and Reauthorization Act, SARA) requires companies to report hazardous chemicals on site to local fire authorities; the public may also request this information. Obviously, once such information is obtained by the local community, local political pressures may be exerted to alleviate community concerns through such actions as reducing chemical stockpiles and even relocating the company.

The doctrine of full disclosure is an essential feature of the National Environmental Policy Act of 1969 (NEPA)—a Federal law that goes well beyond the range of issues considered by occupational safety and health regulations or standards related to hazardous chemicals and which, in the minds of many, is the first piece of modern American legislation devoted to broad environmental objectives and to the roles and responsibilities of Federal agencies regarding those objectives.

It is NEPA that established the Environmental Impact Assessment (EIA) process among Federal agencies in the United States. While impact assessment is today practiced throughout the world in a variety of forms and is the subject of seemingly endless technical, scientific, and political debate, it is worth noting that, in the United States, its primary objective is to improve decision-making by Federal agencies that may influence what (though worded slightly differently from contemporary international pronouncements) is today globally referred to as *sustainable development*. With its emphasis on improved governmental decision-making, the primary means for achieving this goal is a full public disclosure of the environmental issues and concerns addressed (or omitted!) by responsible decision-makers.

It should be noted that the EIA process under NEPA does not include any formal approval process (as, for example, in Malaysia and some other nations). Full disclosure is the means of promoting a public and intra-agency debate. It is this debate and its political repercussions that ultimately determine the final outcome of an agency's proposals for new projects.

Among jurisprudes, NEPA very quickly established itself as an "environmental full disclosure law" and, as such, is viewed as essentially consonant with a more than 300-year and still expanding tradition of Anglo-American jurisprudence of opening governmental decision-making to public scrutiny. In this sense, NEPA as well as many state versions, which are generally known as "environmental acts," are part of an American tradition that also includes the Freedom of Information Act, which is certainly not known as an environmental act.

Within 5 years of its enactment, NEPA was the major statute invoked in environmental litigation, being cited 10 times more often than any other environmental law. Even within such a short period after its implementation, Federal courts interpreted NEPA to establish "substantive rights" and therefore assumed the duty to consider the actual merits of an agency's choice to implement projects. The courts thus went well beyond those traditional rules of American Administrate Law under which the court historically restricted itself to considering simply an agency's procedural correctness.

Significantly, the Federal courts also quickly moved to expand the legal doctrine of "standing," thereby extending the right to sue to conservation groups and other nongovernmental organizations that would not have had court access under traditional rules of court procedures.

It is generally appreciated that the primary strength of NEPA is the simple fact that it so quickly became the basis of a substantial body of case law. Some suggest that the Federal courts actually welcomed NEPA as a means (or excuse) of establishing new precedents. This is, of course, a matter of long-standing debate in the United States regarding the function of the judicial branch of government in "discovering the law" or "making new law" and its consequent role relative to the legislative branch.

In light of these considerations of NEPA, it is reasonable to suggest that the very beginning of modern environmentalism in the United States began not with highly detailed, meticulously defined, scientifically circumscribed environmental objectives but, rather, with the legal empowerment of the public, individual governmental agencies, and nongovernmental organizations (NGOs) to utilize both the judicial system and the court of public opinion on behalf of their environmental concerns. It is this same empowerment that is so important in promoting compliance with the detailed design and performance standards that have since been established.

There can be no doubt whatsoever that the doctrine of full disclosure has resulted in economically wasteful litigative expenditures as well as delays in achieving specific environmental objectives—both in the workplace and the more inclusive human and natural environment. However, it must also be said with equal certainty and, perhaps, with a vigor engendered by a practical appreciation of the difficulties attendant to any social change that, in the absence of both statutory and judicial willingness to implement the doctrine of full disclosure, it is unlikely that environmentalism would have become anything more in the United States than an intellectual hula-hoop or some other essentially banal fad.

The fact remains that the rather tortuous, legal, often overcomplicated, and politically demanding (and frequently frustrating) history of environmentalism in the United States over the past 25 years does seem to have resulted in real and important environmental gains. Our air and water are significantly cleaner than they were; our workplaces are safer; our physical, ecological, archaeological, and historical resources are receiving more attention and care than they formerly received.

More importantly, we are approaching the maturation of that first generation of Americans born and raised in a social, political, economic, and legal milieu in which the word environment connotes not only entrepreneurial and professional opportunity but also a deepening sense of personal and corporate responsibility.

This is not to say that our society is yet mature with respect to environmental issues. We have glaring problems that have yet to be addressed adequately or, frankly, addressed at all. As the first "environmental generation" begins to exert its influence, it is vital that all American generations begin to pay serious attention to two issues in particular: the question of environmental equity and the question of political responsibility.

ENVIRONMENTAL EQUITY AND JUSTICE

If we view the integrated human and natural environment as a source of risk as well as of reward, as the object of human obligations as well as of human rights, and as a place of promise as well as of despair, it is reasonable to ask: Just who takes all the risks, and just who enjoys the rewards? Who has all the obligations, and who has all the rights? Who will be able to realize the promises that begin with every new human life, and who will inherit just the despair? Such questions circumscribe the issue of *environmental equity*—a concern for the socially disproportionate distribution of environmental risks and benefits which, though having been voiced in the United States for over 20 years, has only recently gained significant national as well as international attention.

These questions specifically address the issue of equity because they force consideration of just how benefits and risks are socially distributed with respect to the diverse dimensions of social status, including race, ethnicity, gender, age, and income. They are not sufficient, however, to guide consideration of the more difficult issue of *environmental justice*, a concept that cannot be easily separated from both historical and still developing principles and aspirations regarding the moral and ethical foundations of (and the political responsibility implicit in) any publicly condoned social action—principles, aspirations, and responsibilities that, regardless of how specific consequences of actions undertaken in the name of the public may be distributed within society, would (or should) cause us to consider the worthiness or rightfulness of those actions.

As most commonly used, environmental justice presumes environmental equity—but, more than this, it presumes certain rights of any human regardless of any measure of social status, among which are the rights to a safe, healthful, and nurturing environment. Patterns of environmental inequity or injustice that, regardless of intent, persistently correlate with race may reasonably be (and certainly have been) ascribed to *environmental racism*.

When conducted most rigorously, impact assessment under NEPA requires consideration of the possible impacts of proposed projects on both the physical environment, which most of us perceive and understand as the world of nature, and the social environment. In such a comprehensive approach, impacts on trees and forest are considered, along with impacts on people and communities; impacts on wildlife habitat as well as impacts on human domiciles and neighborhoods; economic impacts as well as ecological impacts. Given such a broad view of assessment, one might presume that the concern for environmental equity and justice has long since been integrated into (and therefore accommodated by) the impact assessment process. But has it?

In the United States, NEPA establishes (among others) the following national goals—goals that are directly pertinent to the issue of environmental equity and that are specifically intended to inform the assessment process:

1. Fulfill the responsibilities of each generation as a *trustee of the environment for succeeding generations*;
2. Assure for *all Americans* safe, healthful, productive, and aesthetically and culturally pleasing surroundings;
3. Preserve important historical, cultural, and natural aspects of our national heritage and maintain, where possible, an environment that *supports diversity and variety of individual choice*; and
4. Achieve a balance between population and resource use that will permit high standards of living and *a wide sharing of life's amenities*.

While such objectives may not define the full range of concerns as expressed in the contemporary environmental equity and justice movement, surely they define a clear congressional intent that the assessment process address the social distribution of environmental benefits and risks; it may also be argued that they imply, even if they do not define, a concept of national environmental rights. However, 26 years after Congress enacted NEPA, the President of the United States deemed it necessary to issue an Executive Order (EO 12898; February 11, 1994) that requires each Federal agency to ". . . make achieving environmental justice part of its mission by identifying and addressing, as appropriate, disproportionately high and adverse human health or environmental effects of its programs, policies, and activities on minority populations and low-income populations in the United States. . . ." It would seem that, even after a quarter of a century, we have yet to come to grips with the social ramifications of environmental impacts on humans.

While the ongoing and expanding concern for environmental equity and justice is historically linked in the United States to environmental legislation related to such issues as impact assessment (NEPA), hazardous waste management (Resource Conservation and Recovery Act, RCRA), and clean water and air (Clean Water Act, CWA; Clean Air Act, CAA), environmental equity and justice are equally relevant to the issue of health and safety in the workplace which, after all, is not only a significant environment to employees for a substantial portion of their time, but also the potential source of contaminants having impact on surrounding environments.

POLITICAL RESPONSIBILITY

The NIMBY (not-in-my-back-yard) syndrome is known throughout the world. However, this does not excuse the persistent American failure to come to grips with the environmental implications of an historical delineation of Federal and states rights or of the differential political empowerment of communities on the basis of race, income, and education.

While American Federal law requires a cradle-to-grave approach to the management of hazardous waste, we have to date no realistic political mechanism to ensure that properly engineered treatment–storage–disposal facilities are located with any sense of geographical balance. In consequence, a few states become the dumping grounds of many states, with not only possible severe consequences to current workers but also to the future generations of Americans in those few states as well as to those human populations potentially exposed during the intrastate transport of wastes.

It is clear that historical political structures are not only inadequate for dealing with current waste-disposal problems, but also exacerbate those problems through various economic competitions among states and the sometimes bewildering plurality of political jurisdictions.

As early as 1967, the U.S. Congress began to deal with jurisdictional aspects of environmental contaminants in its then unique approach to managing air quality—an approach that has continued to be expanded in the more current Air Quality Act. Such creative legislative approaches have yet to be applied to the disposal of hazardous wastes or to the relative risks of workers on the basis of the particular state or region in which they happen to live and work.

In the progress of the as yet nascent social and political debate regarding the implications of environmental equity and justice, it is reasonable to assume that traditional distinctions between the workplace and the environment will become more broadly seen as arbitrary in the sense that such distinctions are probably reflective more of the particular historical development of legal, commercial, and political institutions than of any overpowering pragmatic logic or empirical necessity. In such a circumstance, it may well be considered that the workplace is as rightfully subject to the standard of equitable justice as any other resource that contributes to the total human environment. Certainly, the likelihood that such a consideration will receive significant social and political attention is only to be increased by the ongoing cultural diversification of the American workforce, the persistent concern of the American public regarding human health and the quality of life, and the proliferation of global enterprise.

THE GLOBAL CONNECTION

Over the past 25 years of the modern environmental movement, there have been many political changes in the United States, including 6 presidencies and 14 U.S. Congresses. Throughout this period, especially at times of change in political administrations, there has been the usual number of pundits who have predicted that the business community would finally be given relief from the regulatory demands of occupational health and safety and environmental quality regulations. The pundits, of course, have been consistently wrong. They were wrong because they overlooked both the persistency and consistency with which the American public has supported the objectives of human health and environmental quality, even in periods of national economic despair and international turmoil.

It is because of the public demand for governmental action that, quite contrary to the predictions of pundits, regulatory demands have become not only more numerous, but also more complex, more interconnected, and more pervasive throughout American society. The most recent Federal exercise in "reinventing government," whatever its achievements may be, is not likely to reverse this trend or otherwise substantially alter it. Not because there are none who have the political will to do so, nor because there are no good reasons for making changes—but, rather, simply because the stubborn demand of the American public for human health and environmental quality is fundamentally consistent with the growing demands of the global marketplace.

There can be no question that the "greening" of the global economy is infused with the full panoply of competitive machinations and strategies that have ever characterized the social, political, and economic interactions of diverse peoples and interests. Certainly the banner of human health and safety and environmental quality does not signal the demise of self-aggrandizement or avarice; rather, it can become (and perhaps it already has become) itself a rallying flag for these and other vices as well as for virtue.

If there is one fact that must be emphasized about the global marketplace it is that human health and safety and environmental quality objectives have been co-opted by both northern and southern corporations as essential marketing tools, with North American, United European, and Southern Asian nations already poised to implement formal procedures for certifying the authenticity and efficacy of those tools.

Just as the rapid integration of the regulatory objectives of the National Environmental Policy Act into case law served not only to enervate the early environmental movement in the United States but also to preserve it from abrupt political redirection, so might the emergence of human health and safety objectives and environmental quality as practical business strategies similarly function in the international arena—by transforming these objectives into an essential *lingua franca* of a necessarily global economic system.

Of particular importance in this business-driven paradigm of health, safety and environment is the southern insistence, as expressed in the Rio Conference of 1992, that the historically northern compartmentalization of human health and environmental quality be abandoned as an economically inefficient and conceptually untenable academic exercise—that the social and physical environments of humankind cannot be abstracted from one another and must therefore be managed (if managed at all) holistically.

It should be clearly understood that this shift in paradigm directly conflicts with the traditional northern view of the workplace as basically an economic resource to be wielded simply for economic objectives and, as such, essentially immune to the supposed vagaries of any social engineering or tinkering. The vast majority of humankind has decided otherwise and, to the degree that the minority northern nations intend to participate in—and thereby influence—a global economy, the northern nations will find it increasingly necessary to deconstruct the artificial barriers that separate the workplace from an all encompassing human environment.

INDEX